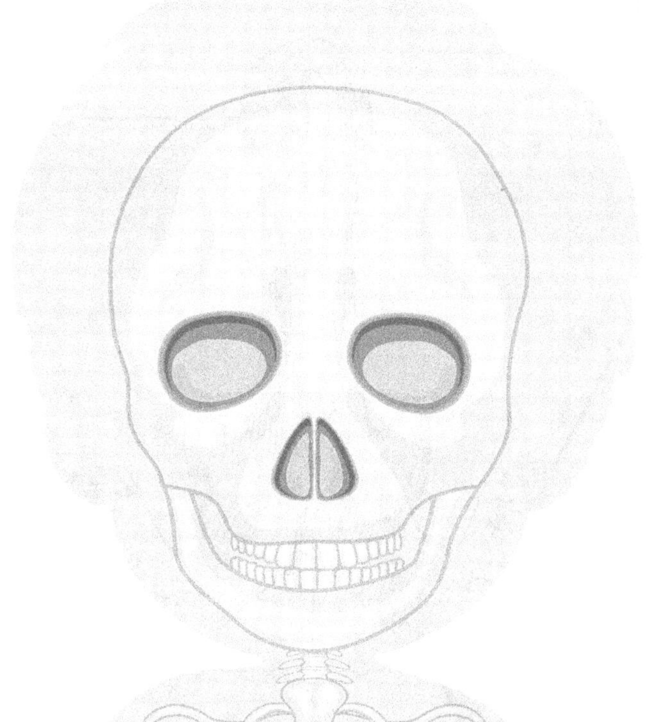

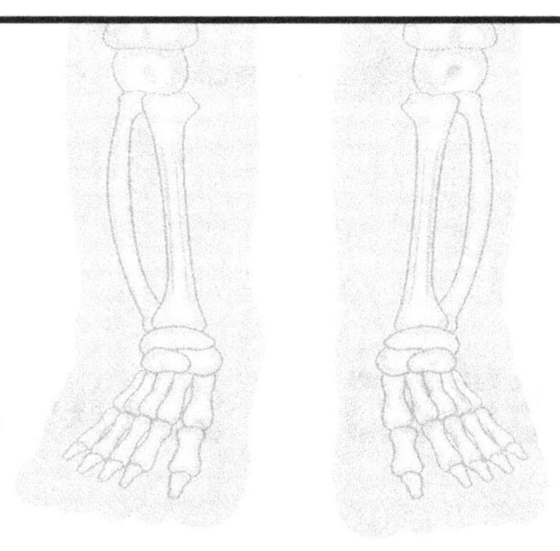

THIS BOOK BELONGS TO

____

____

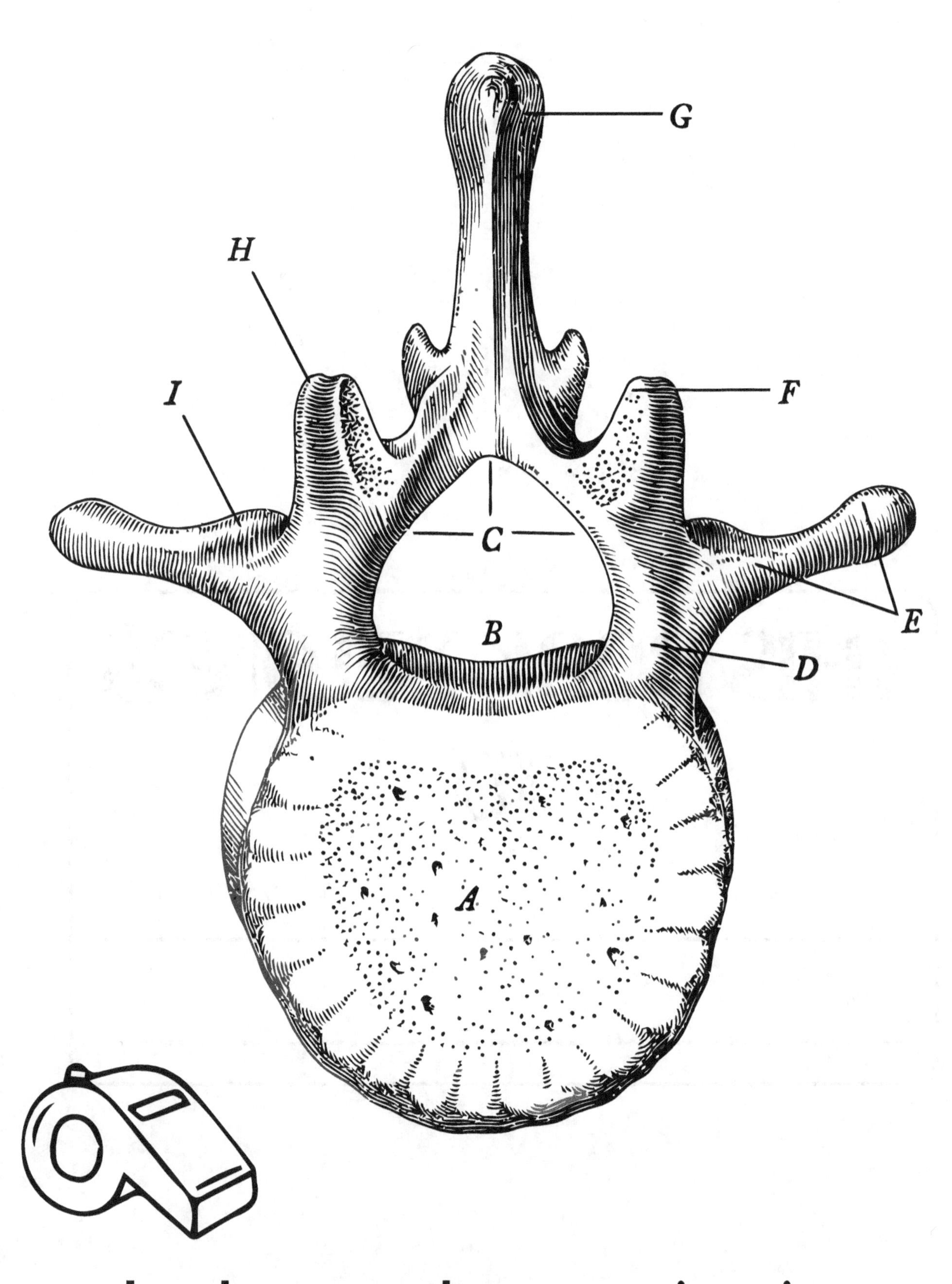

Lumbar vertebra superior view

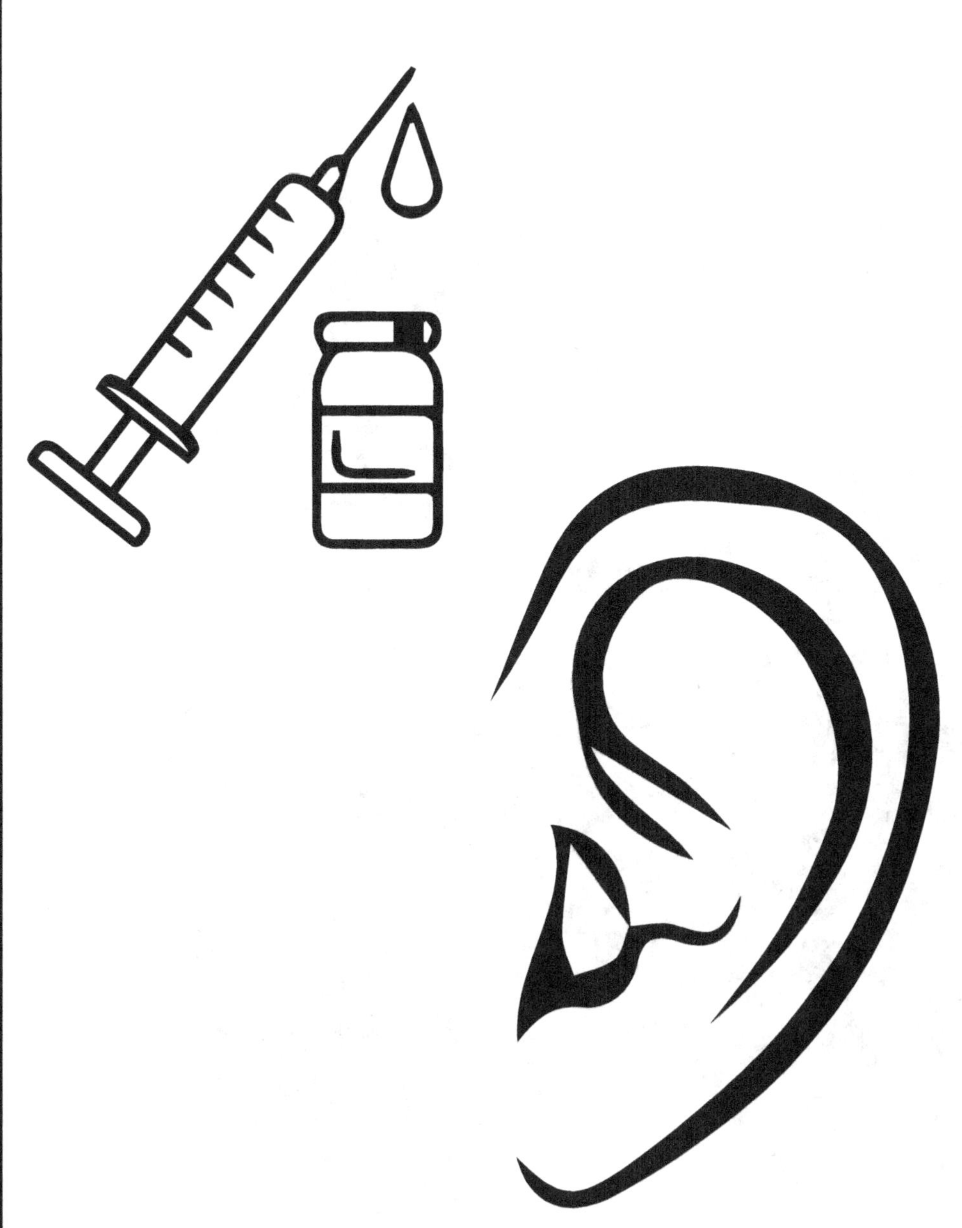

Otolaryngology

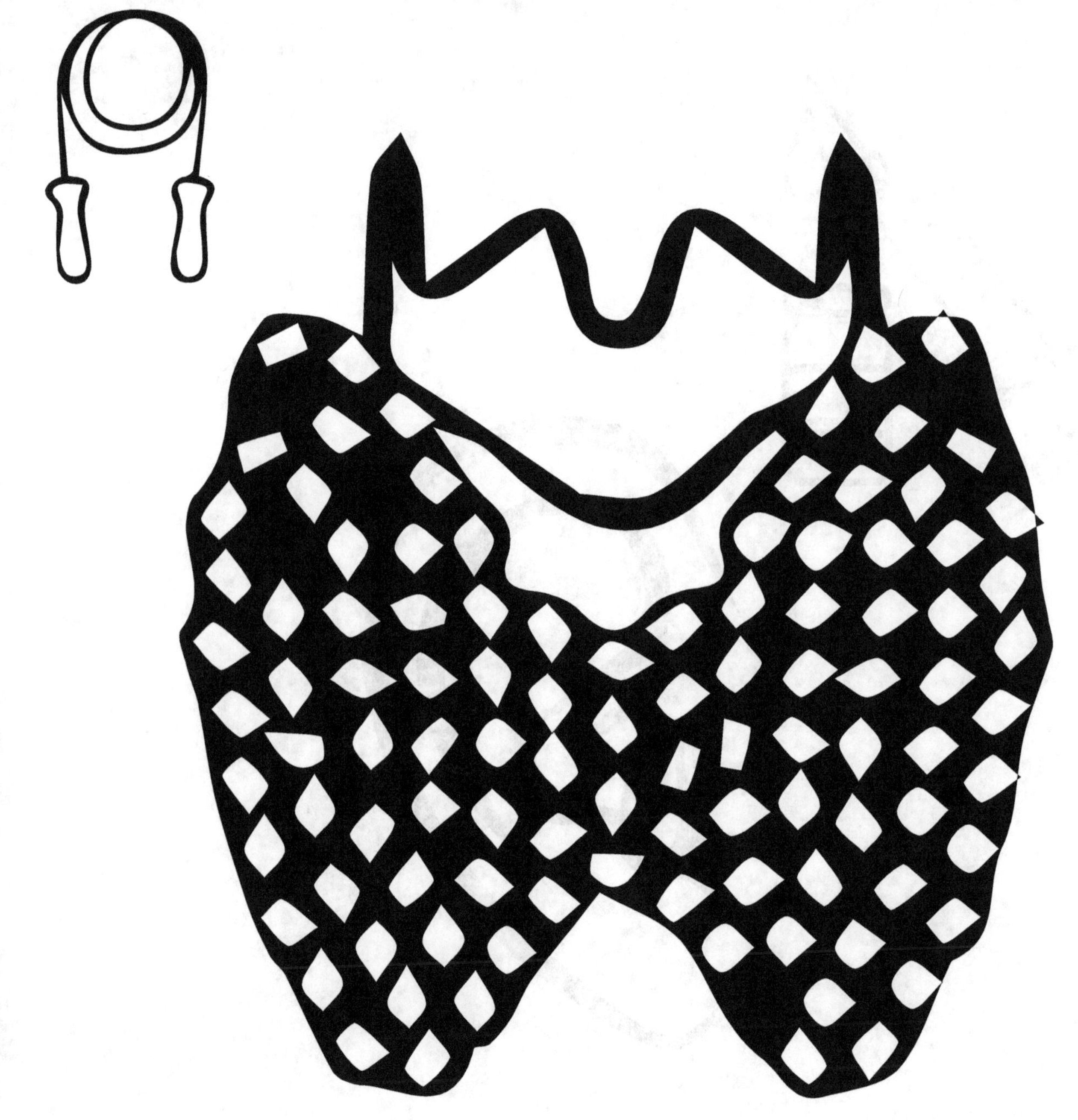

Endocrinology

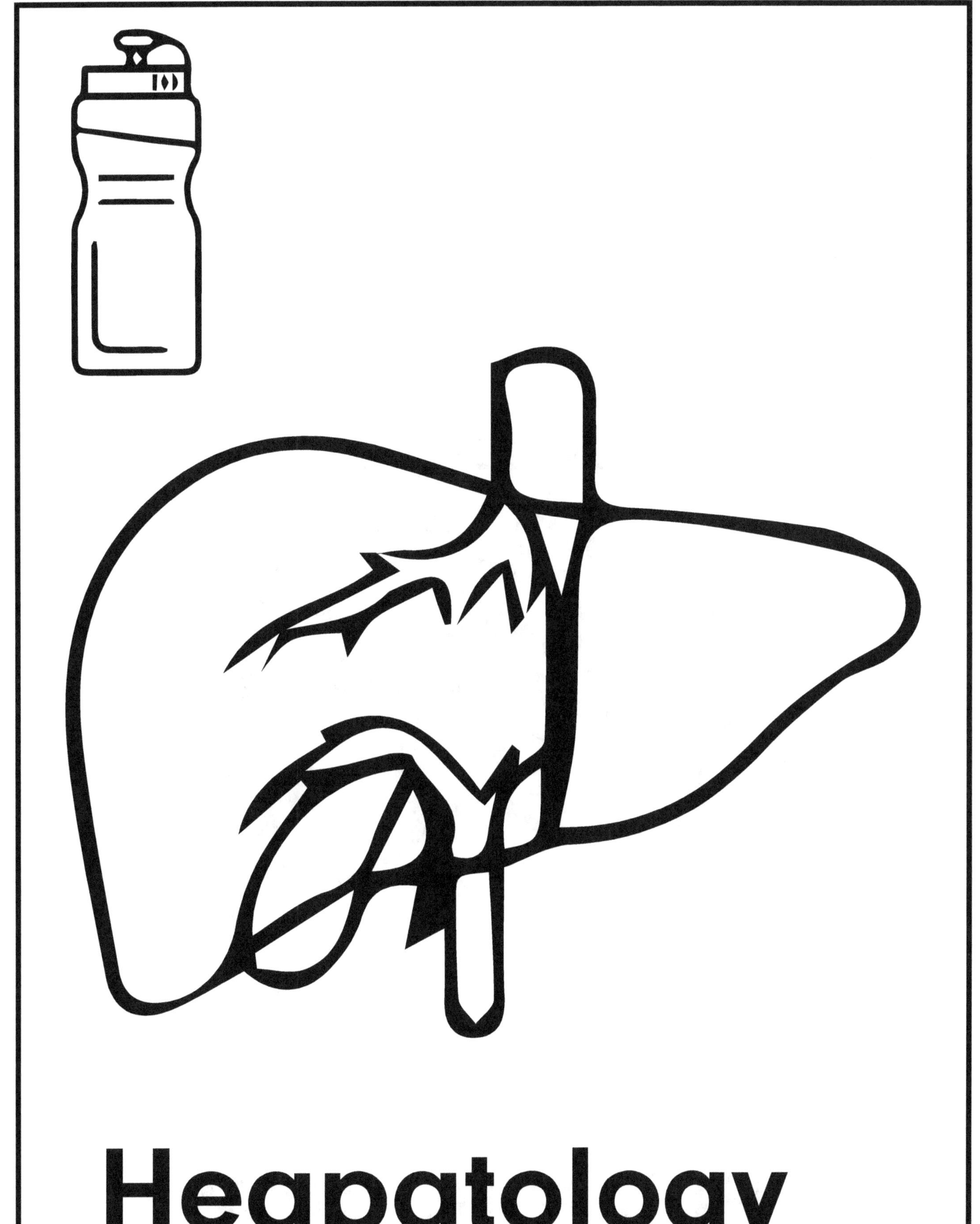

Heapatology

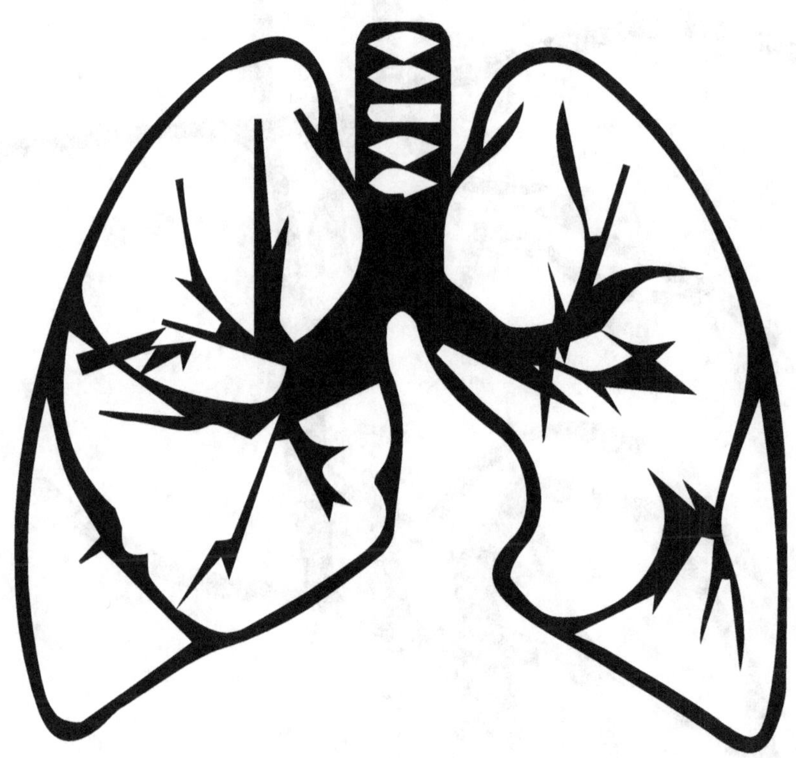

Pulmonology

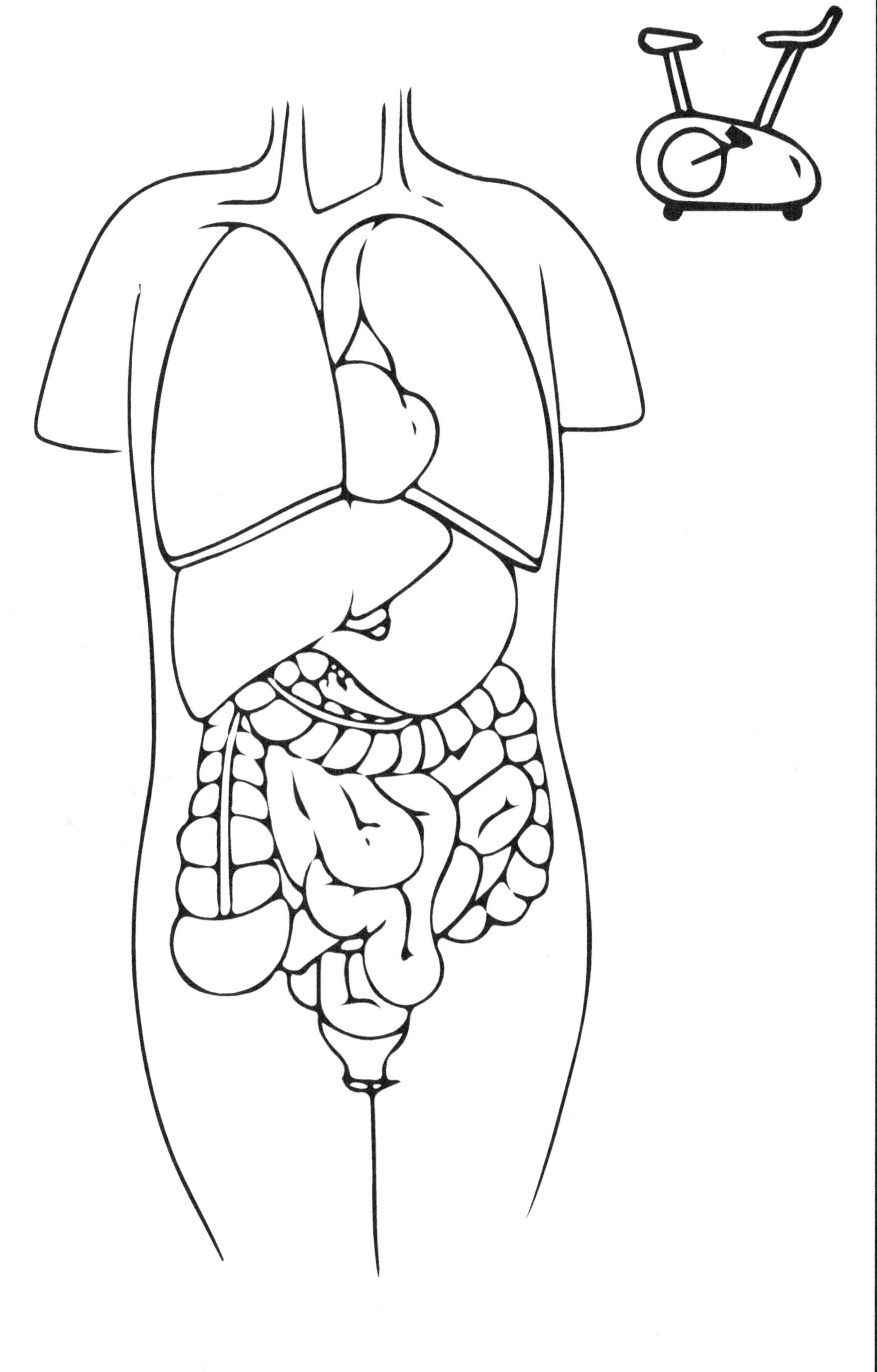

ORGANS STUCTURE

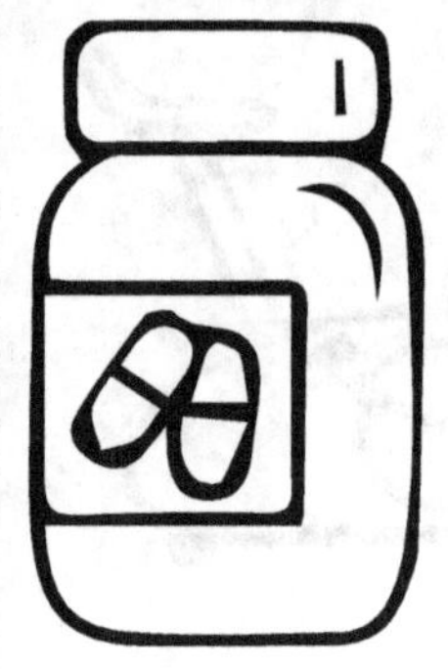

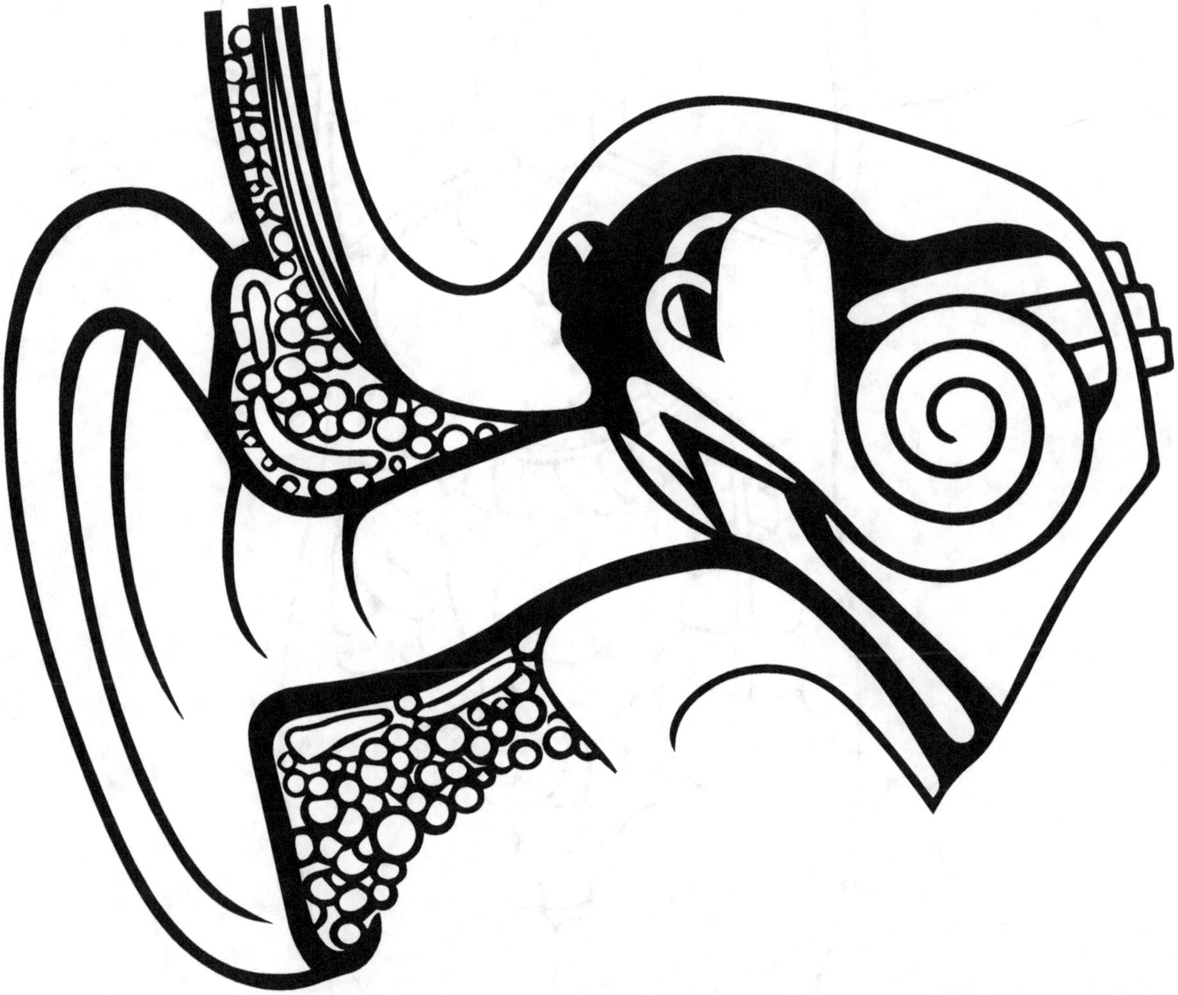

Ear Diagram

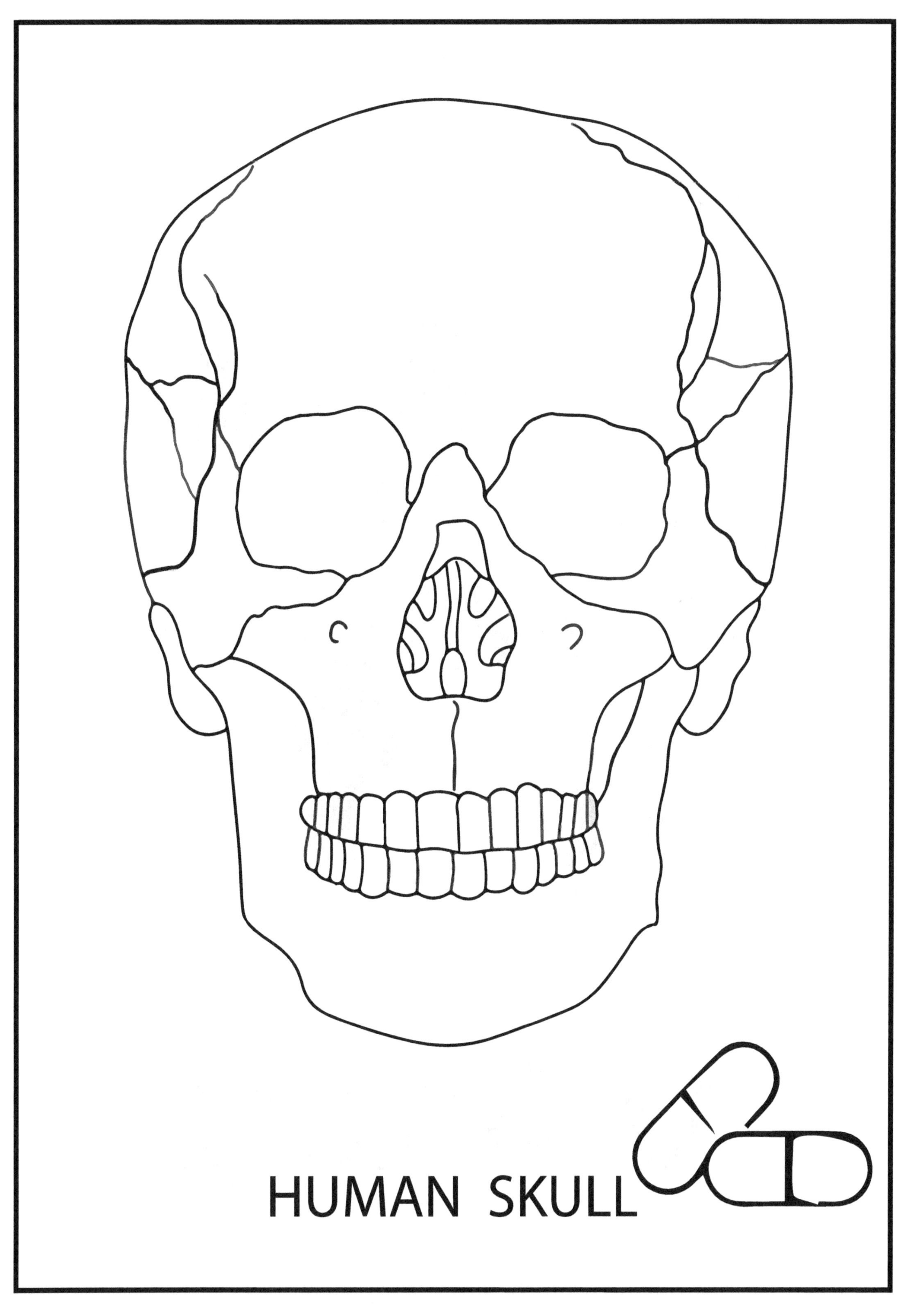

HUMAN SKULL

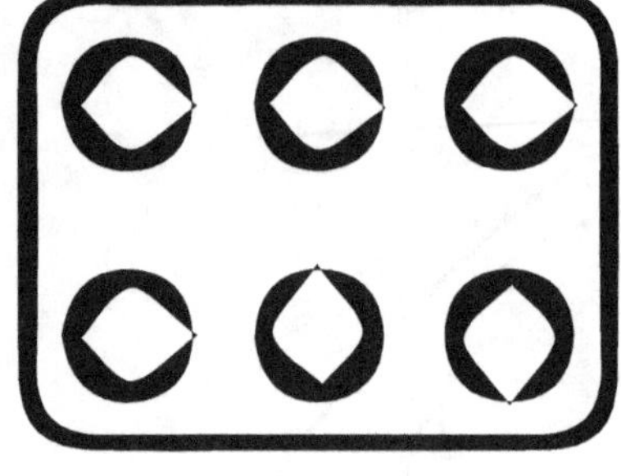

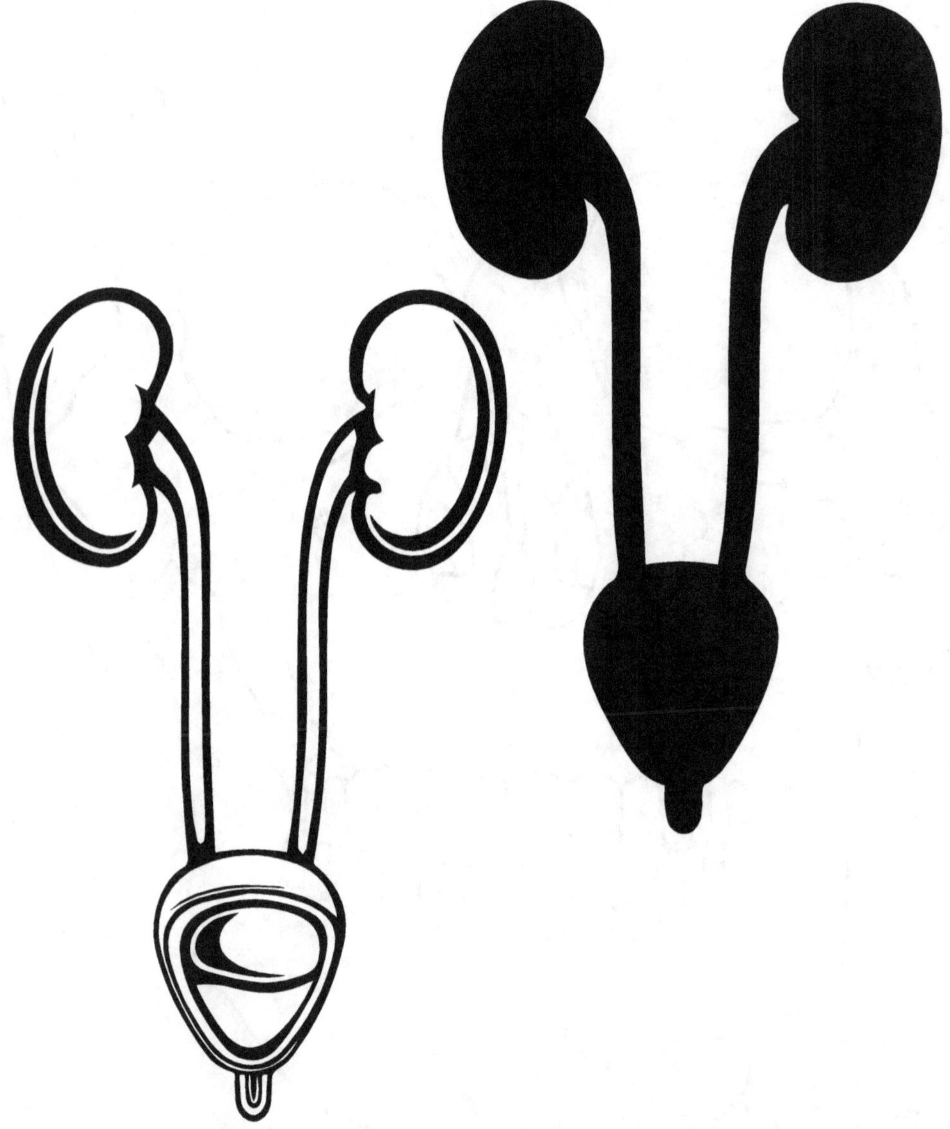

Urinary

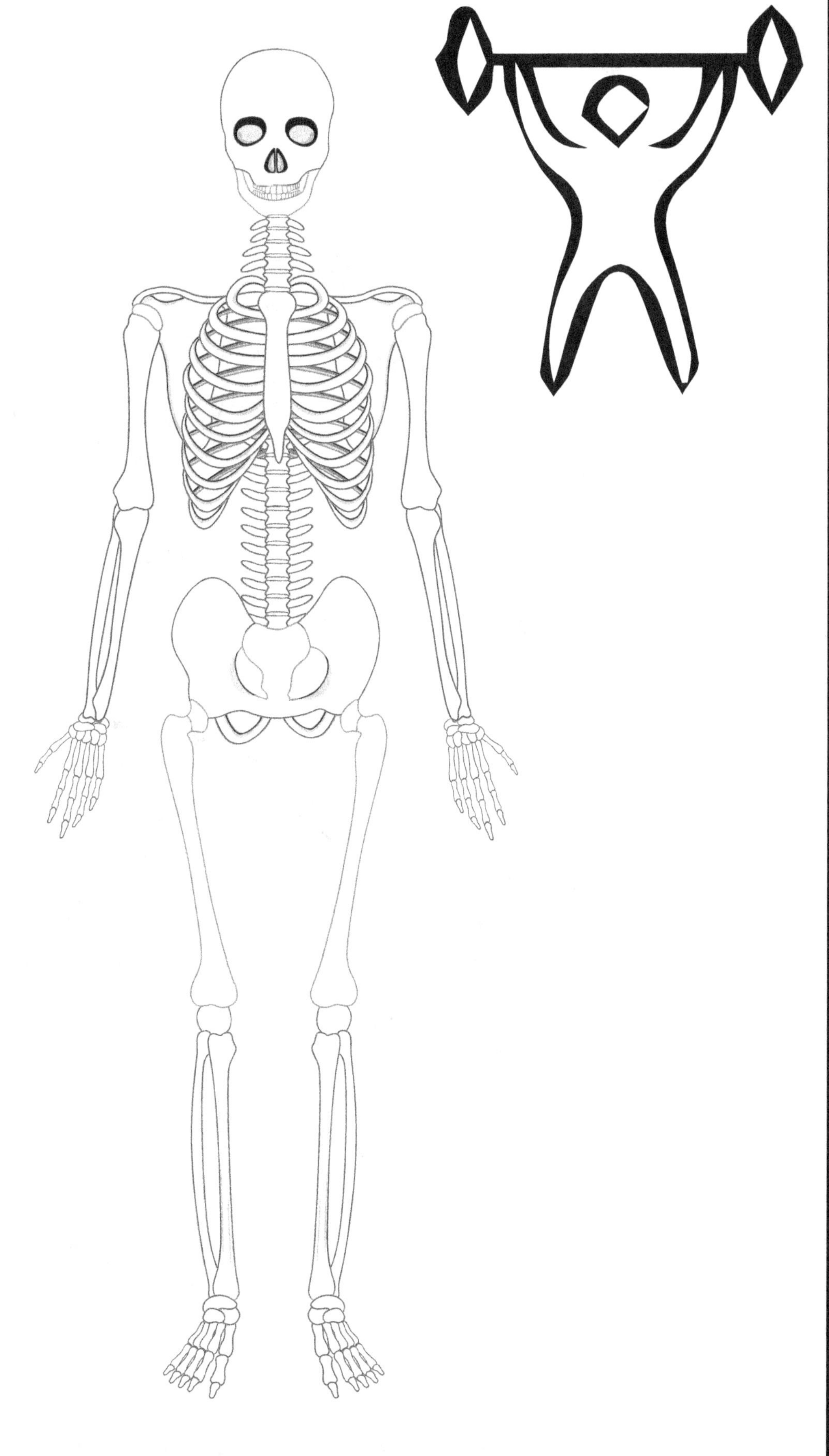

HUMAN SKELETON STRUCTURE

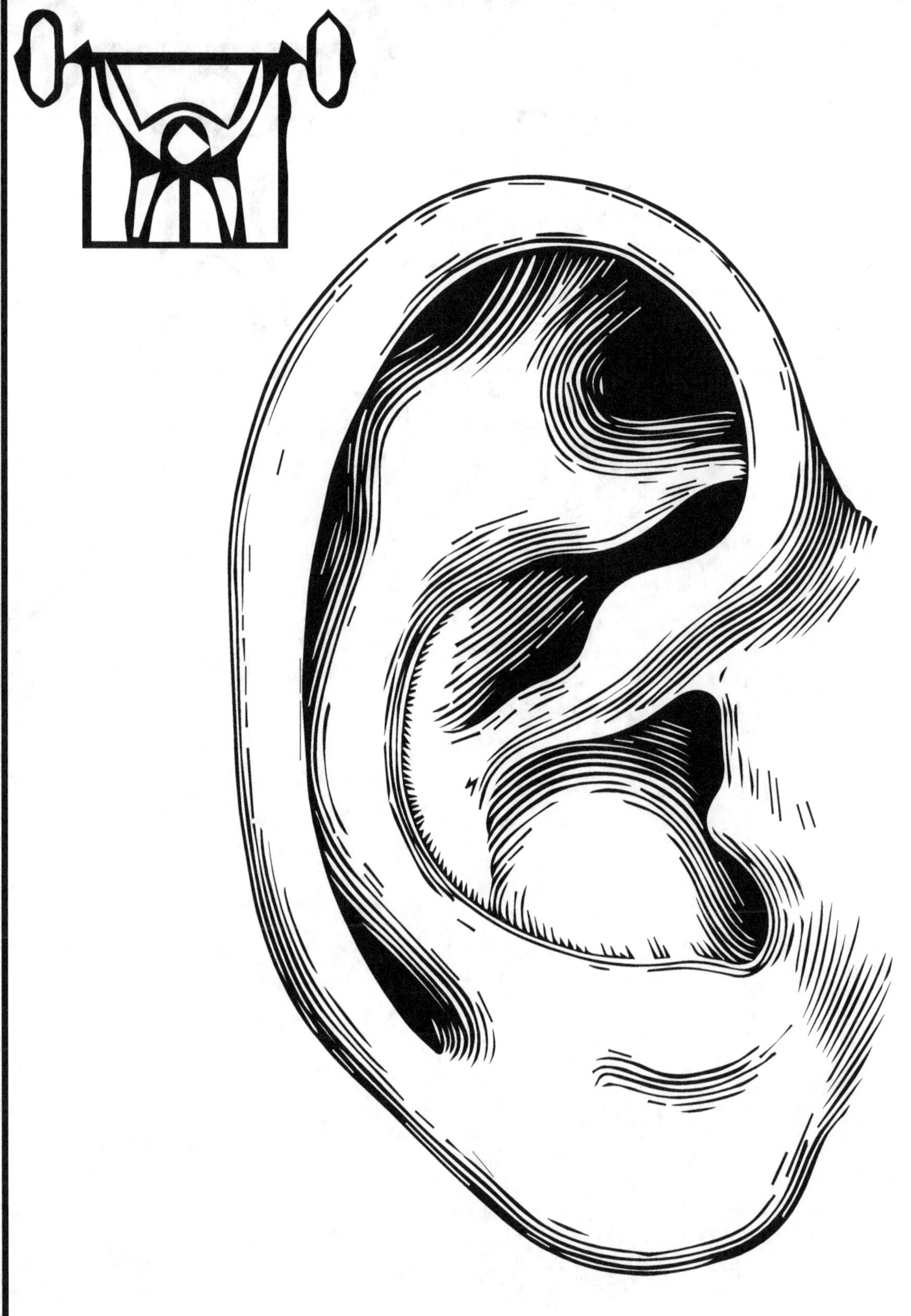

Human ear hand

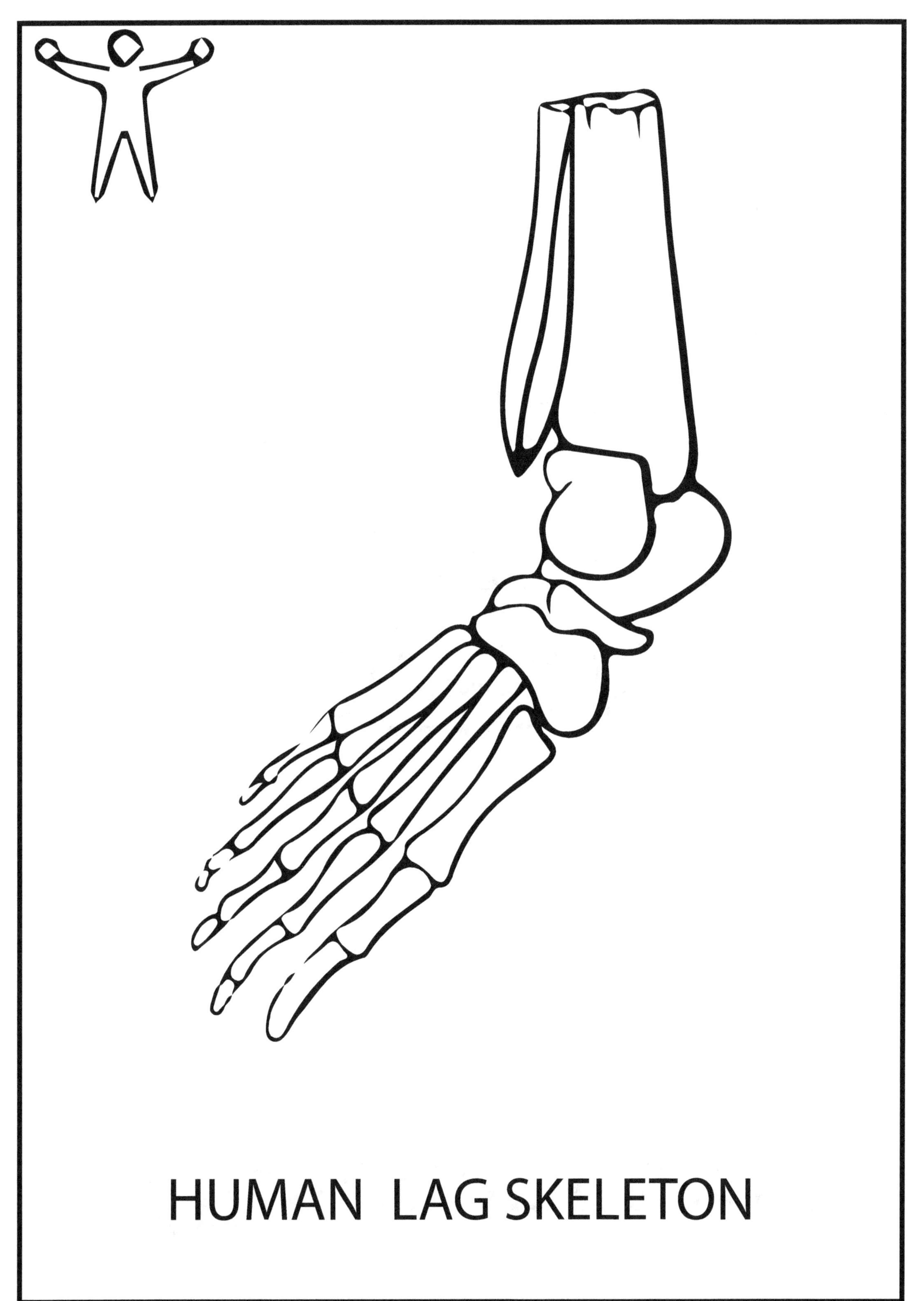

HUMAN LAG SKELETON

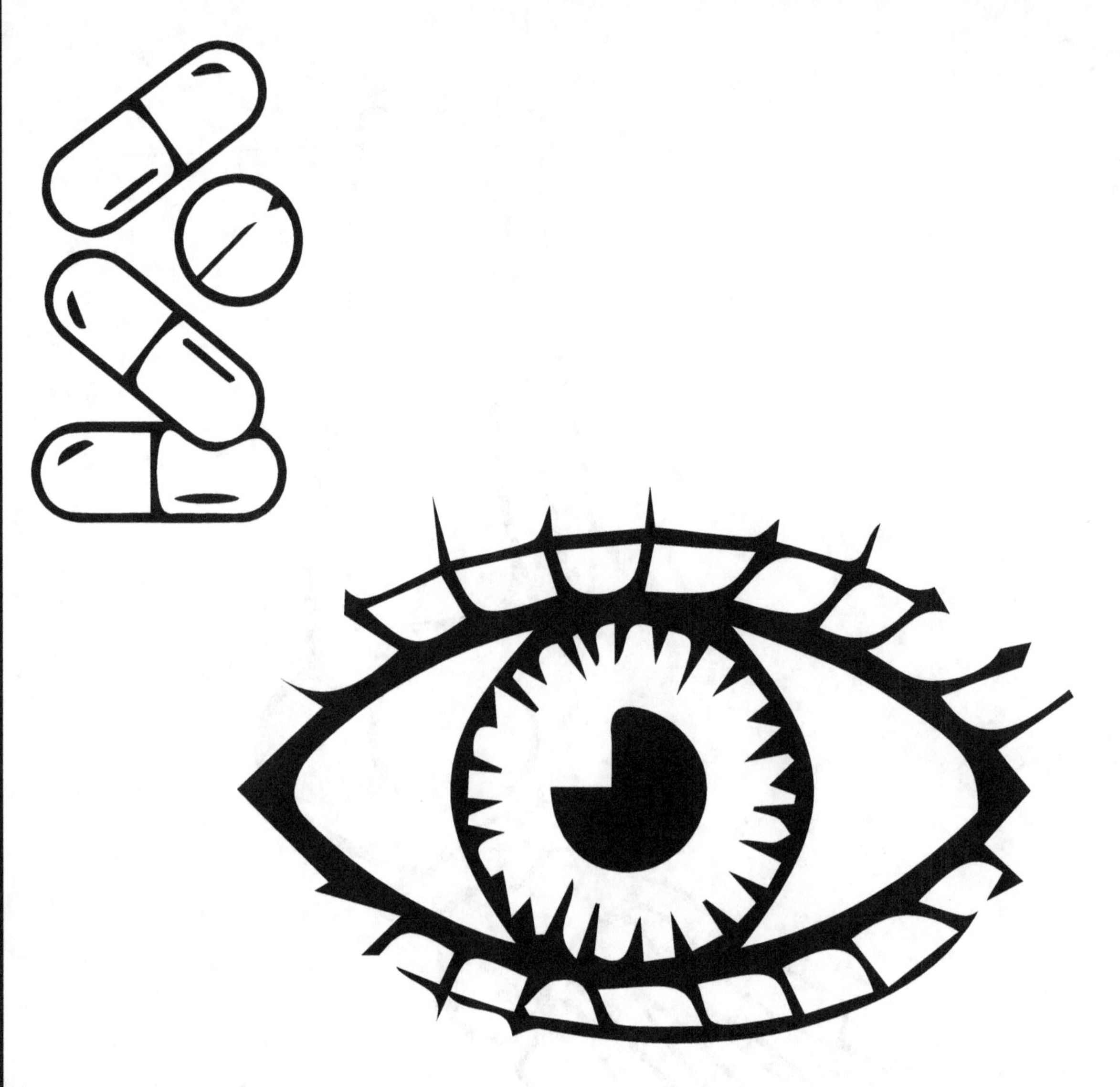

Ophthalmology

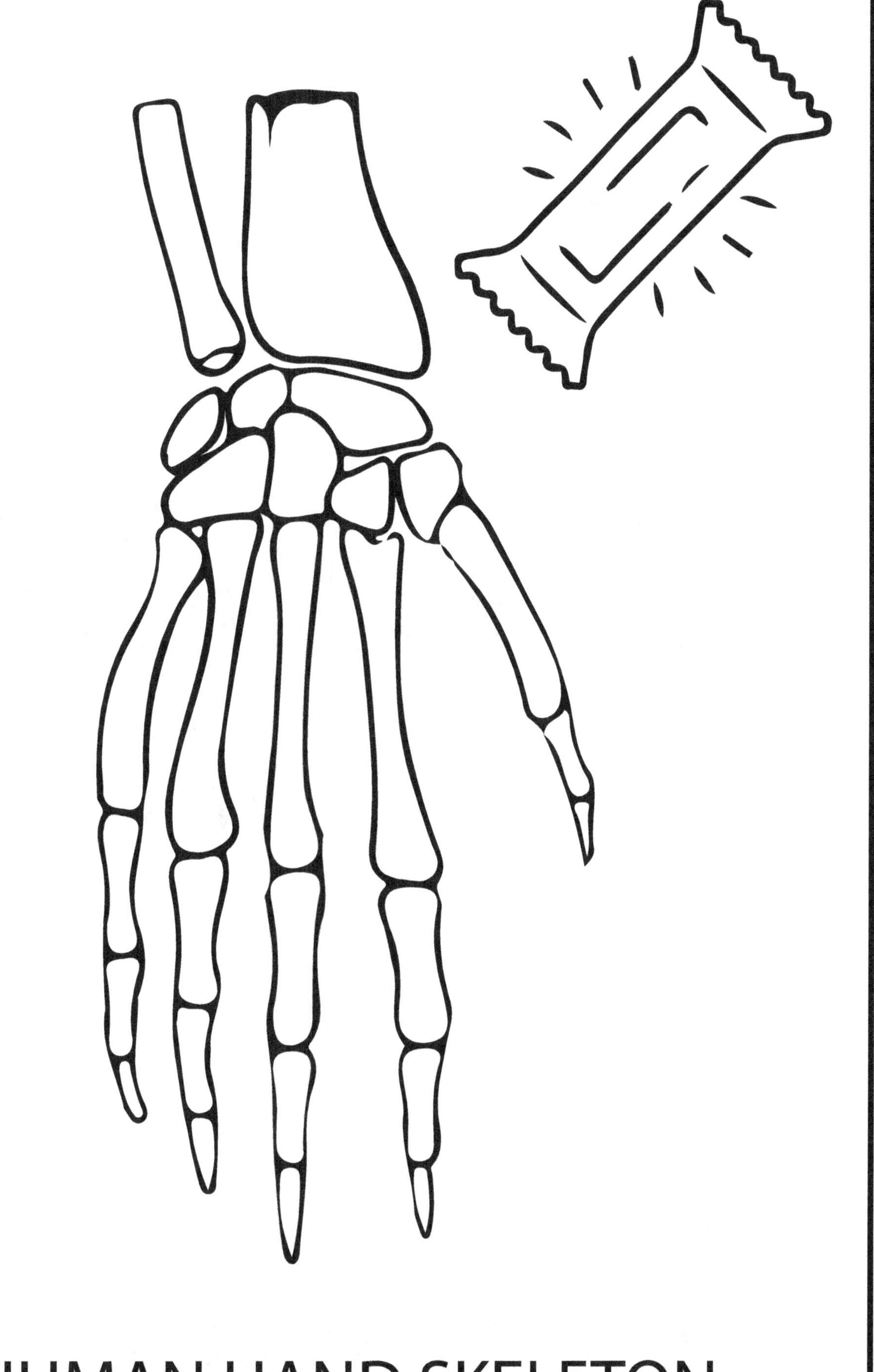

HUMAN HAND SKELETON

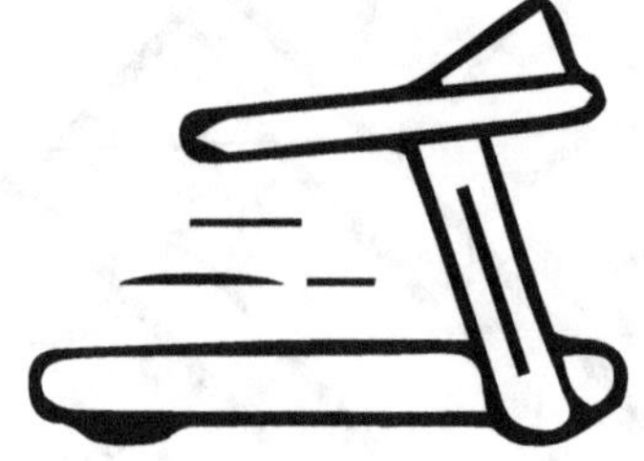

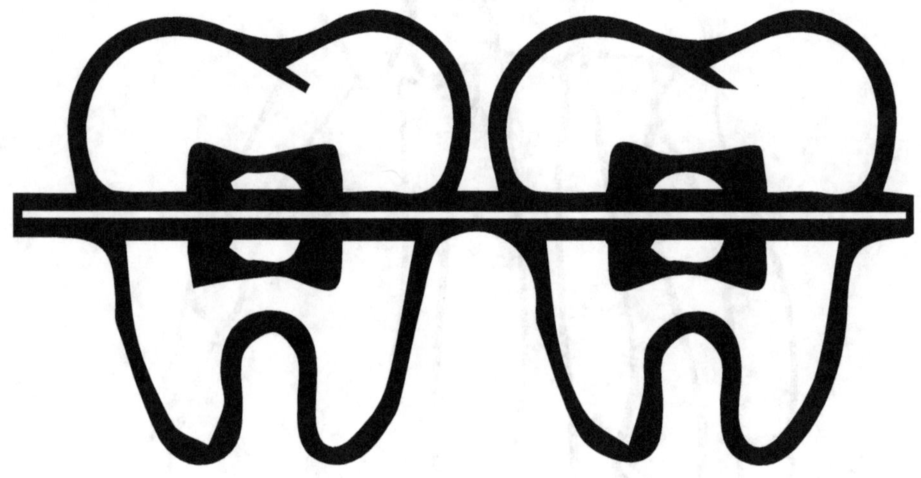

Dentisity

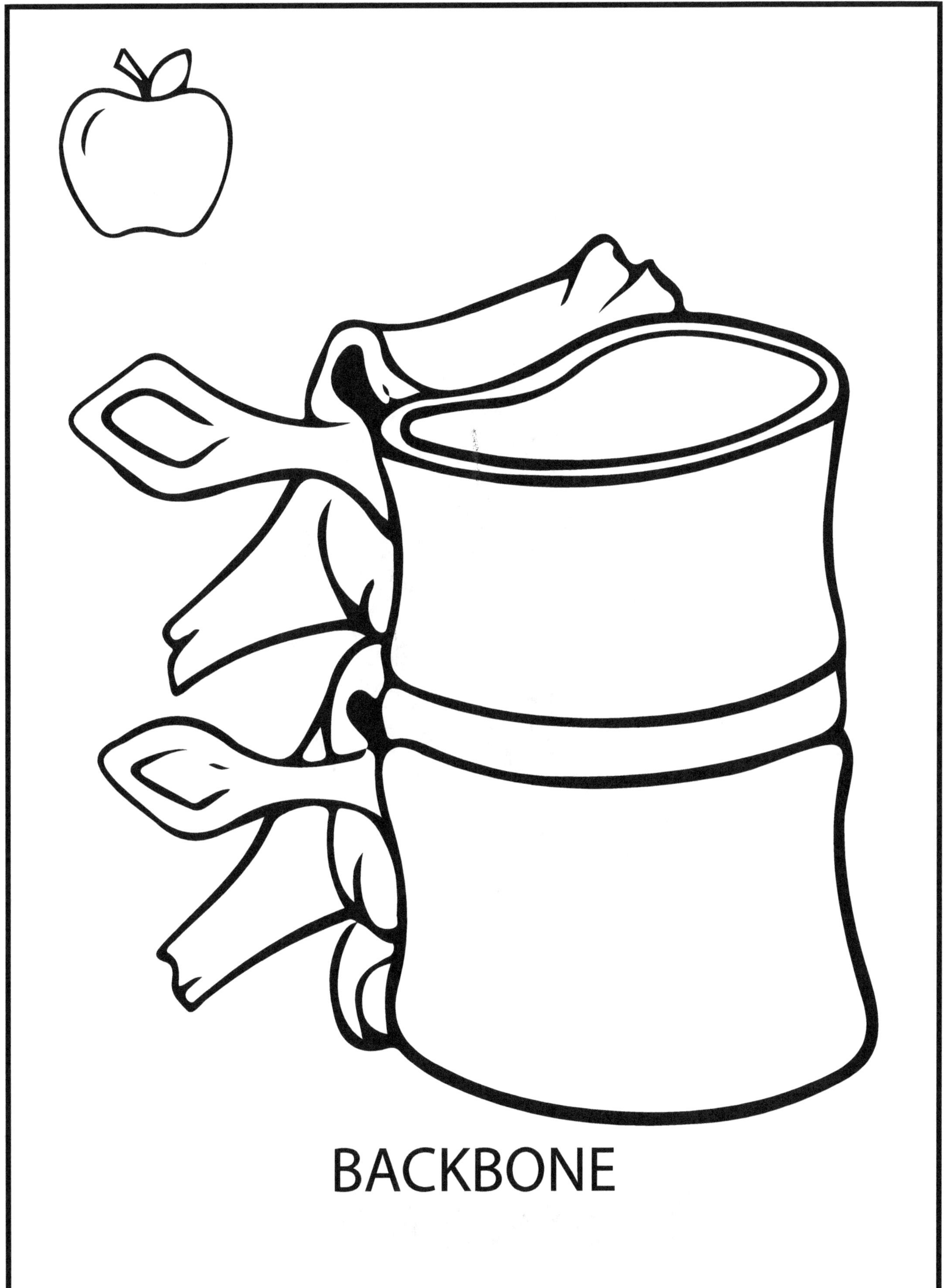

BACKBONE

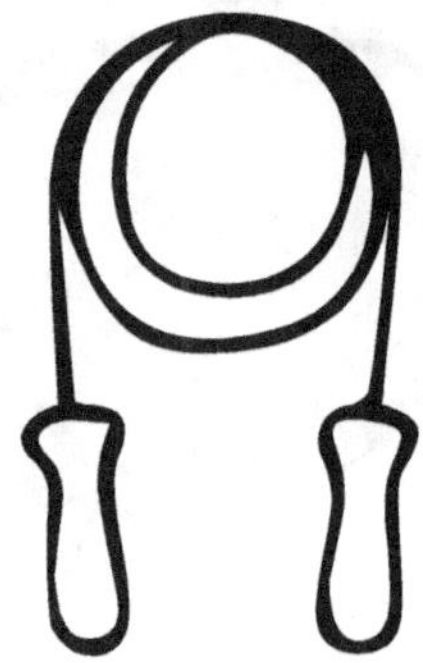

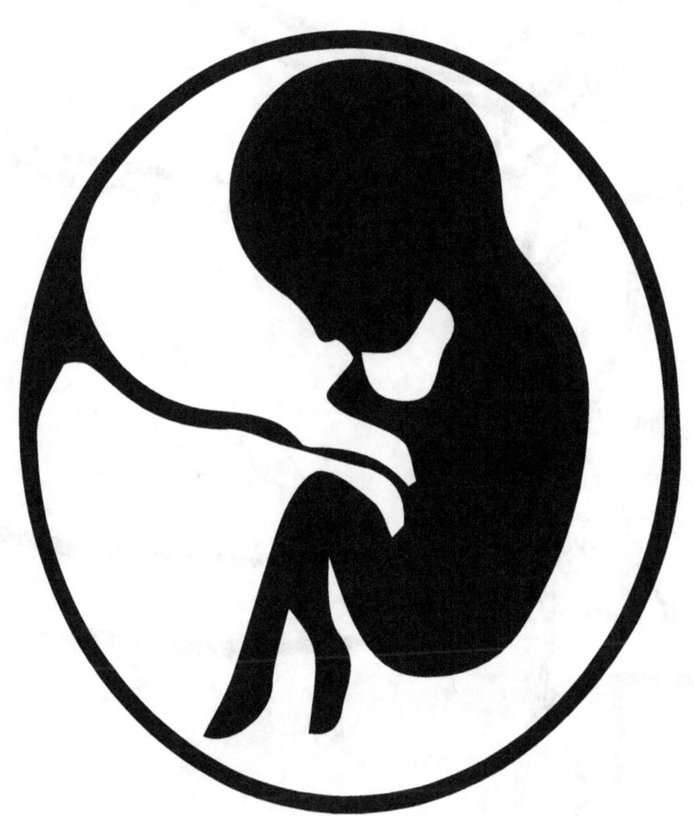

Obstetrics

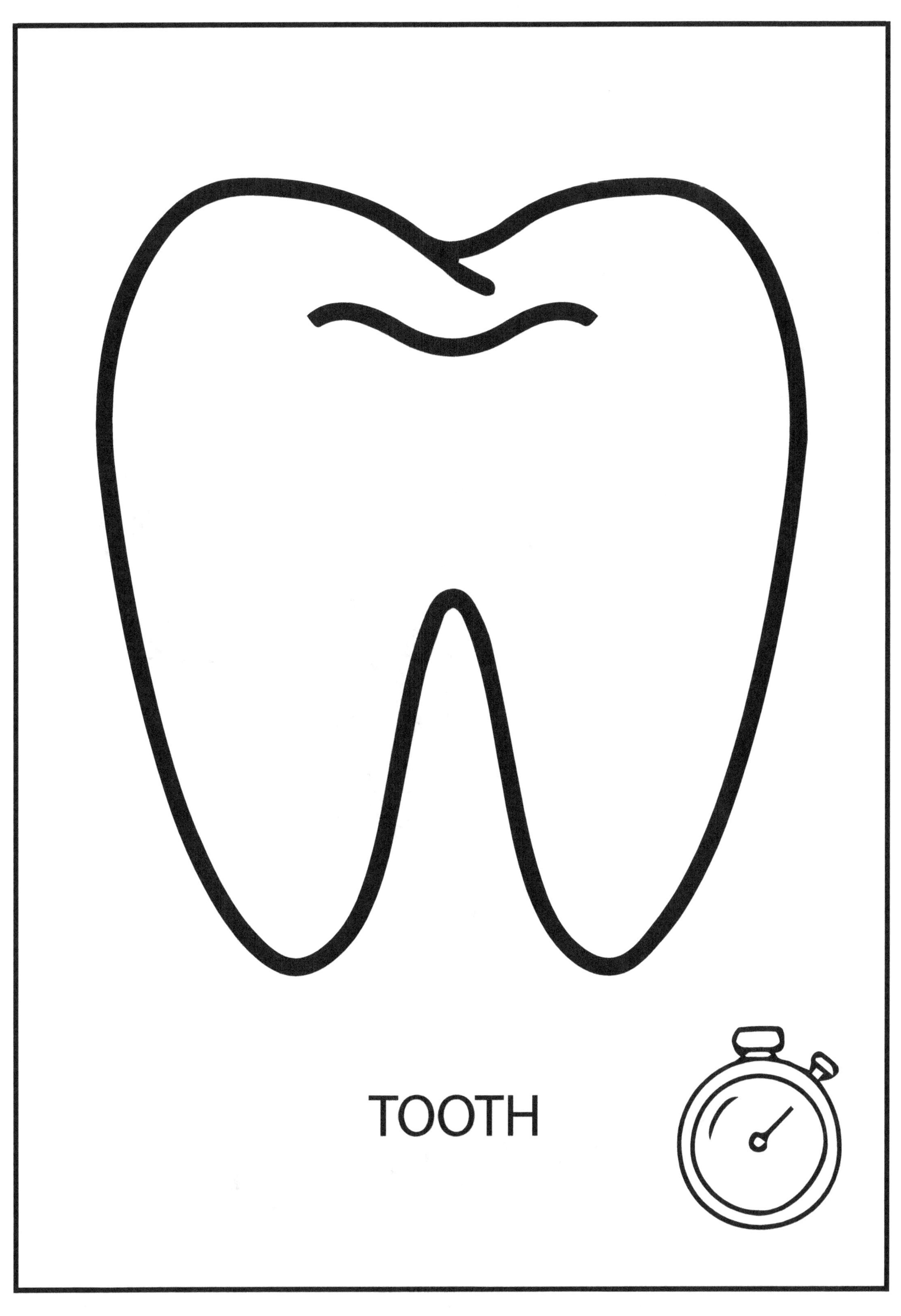

TOOTH

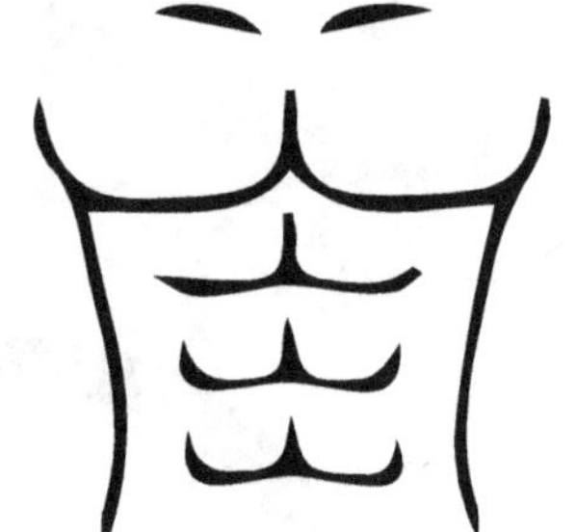

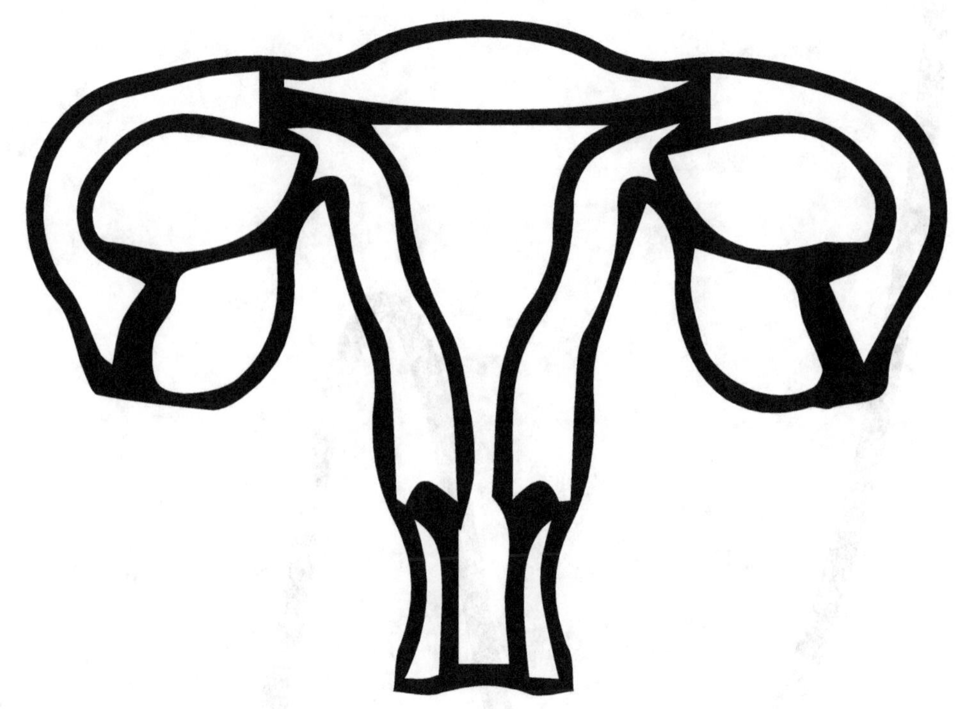

Gynecology

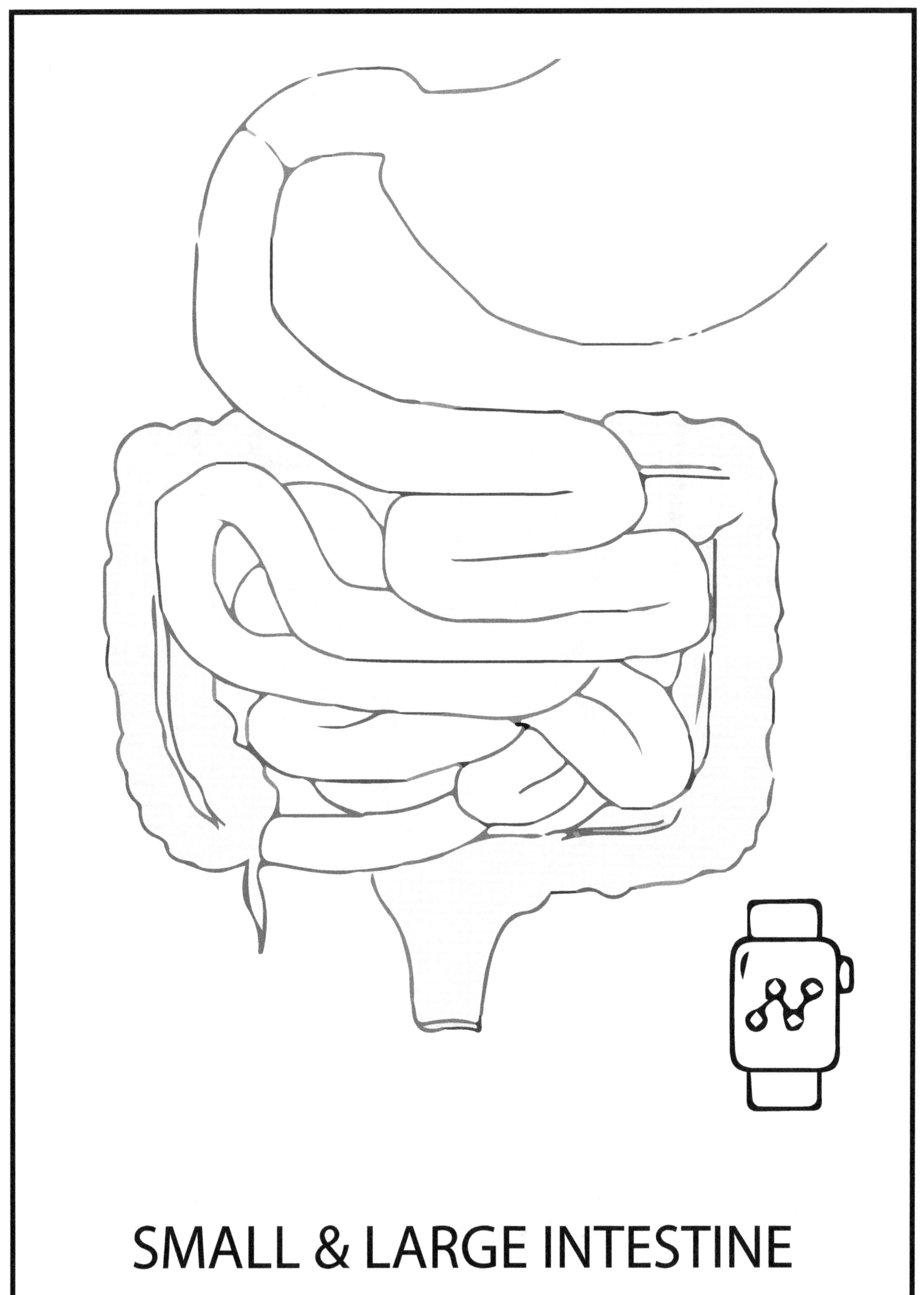

SMALL & LARGE INTESTINE

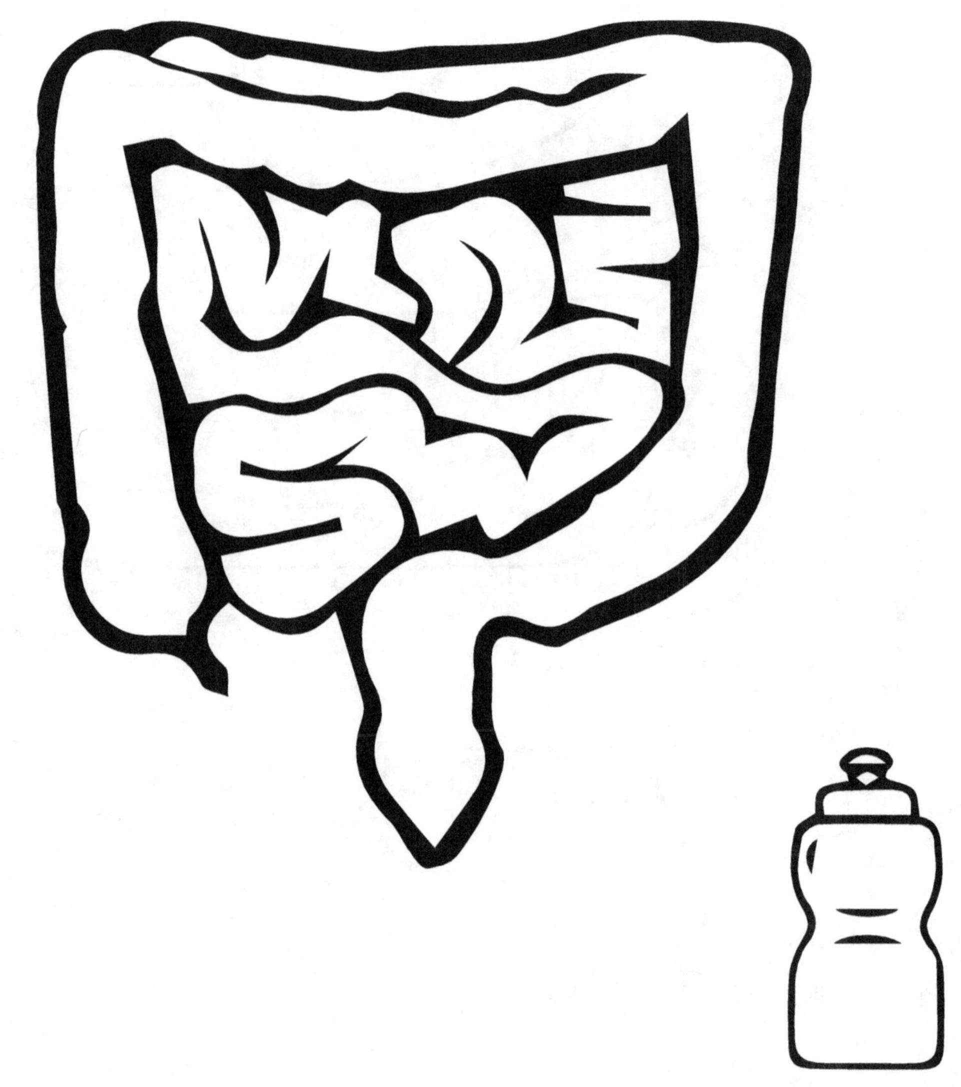

Gastroenterology

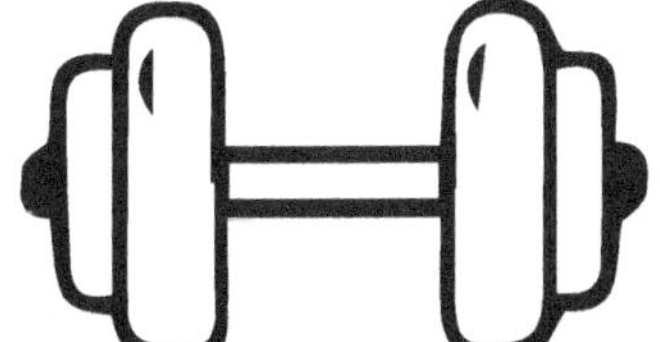

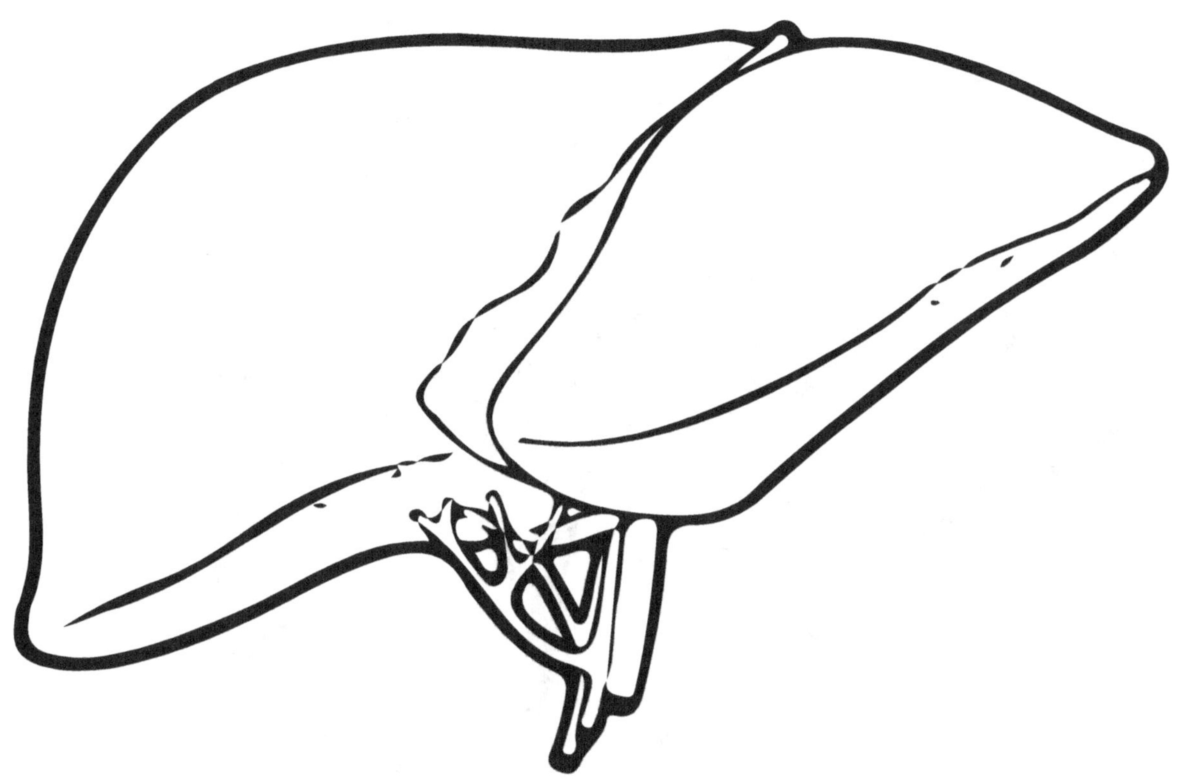

LIVER

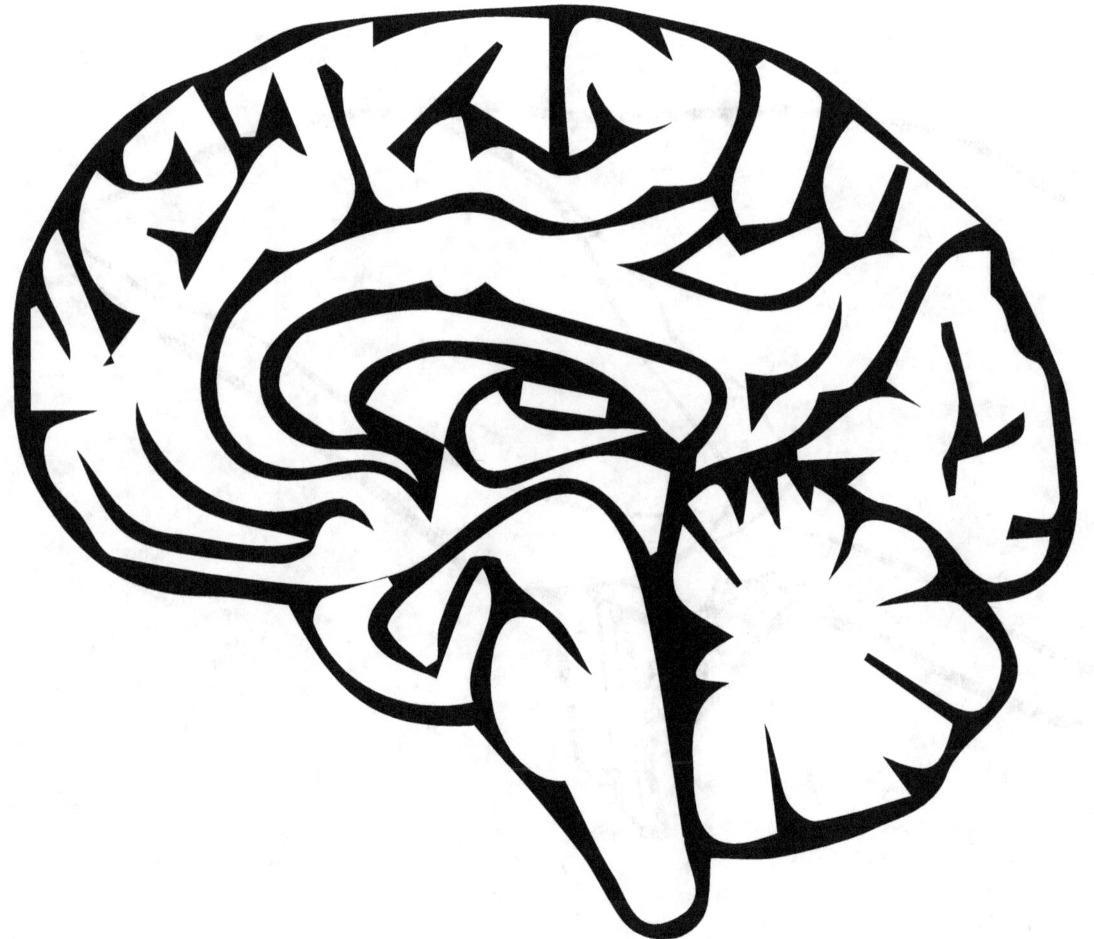

Neurology

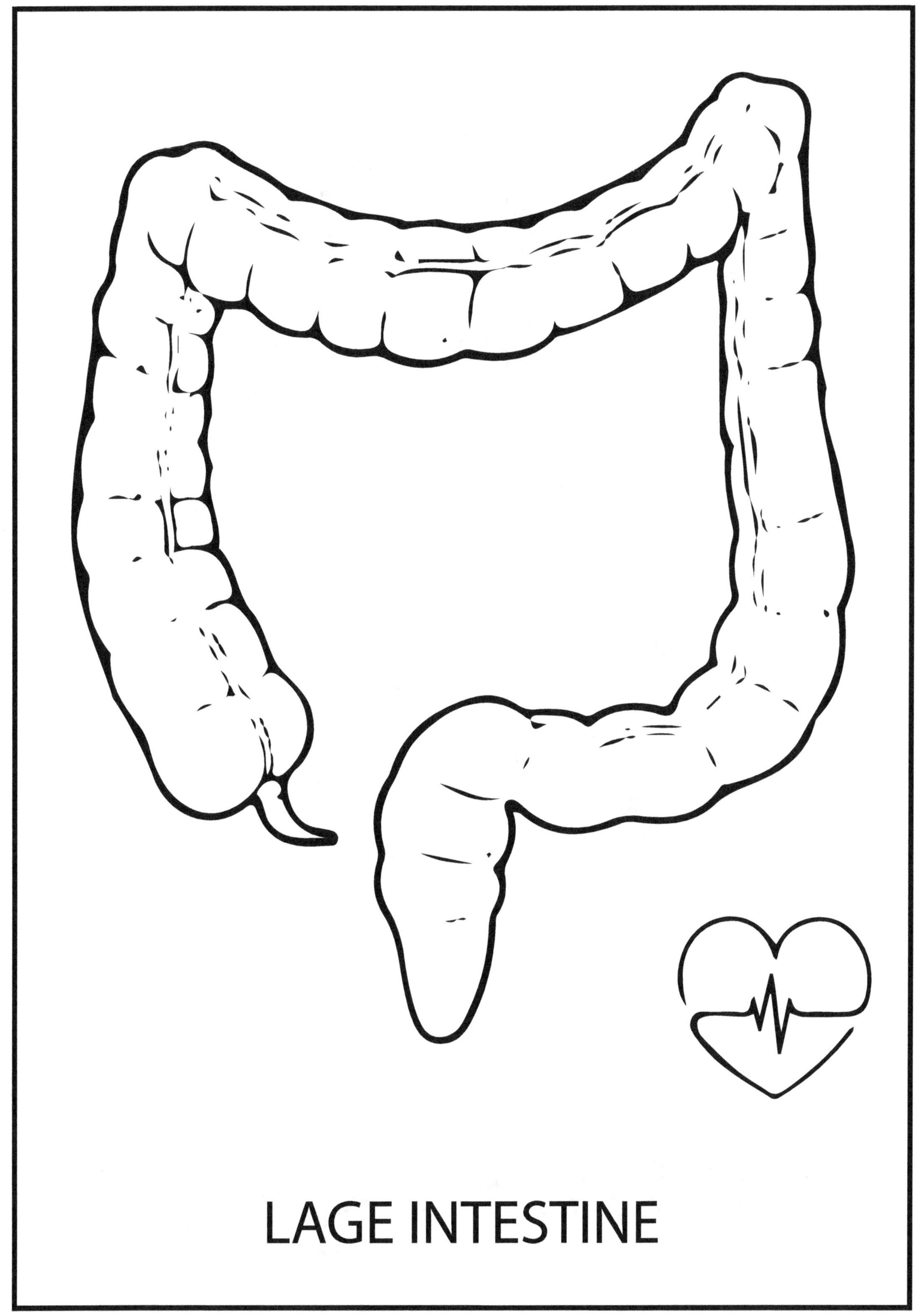

LAGE INTESTINE

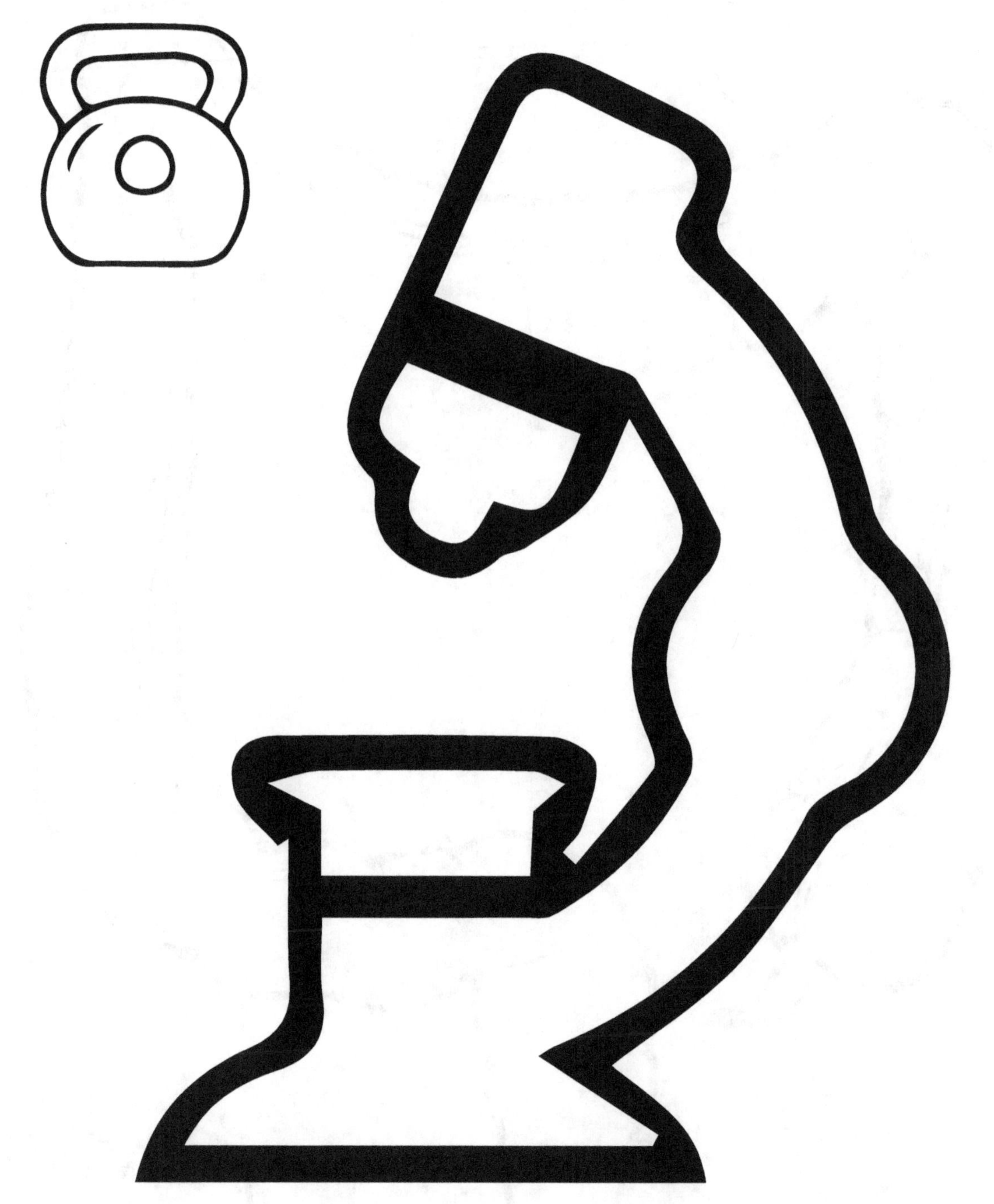

Pathological

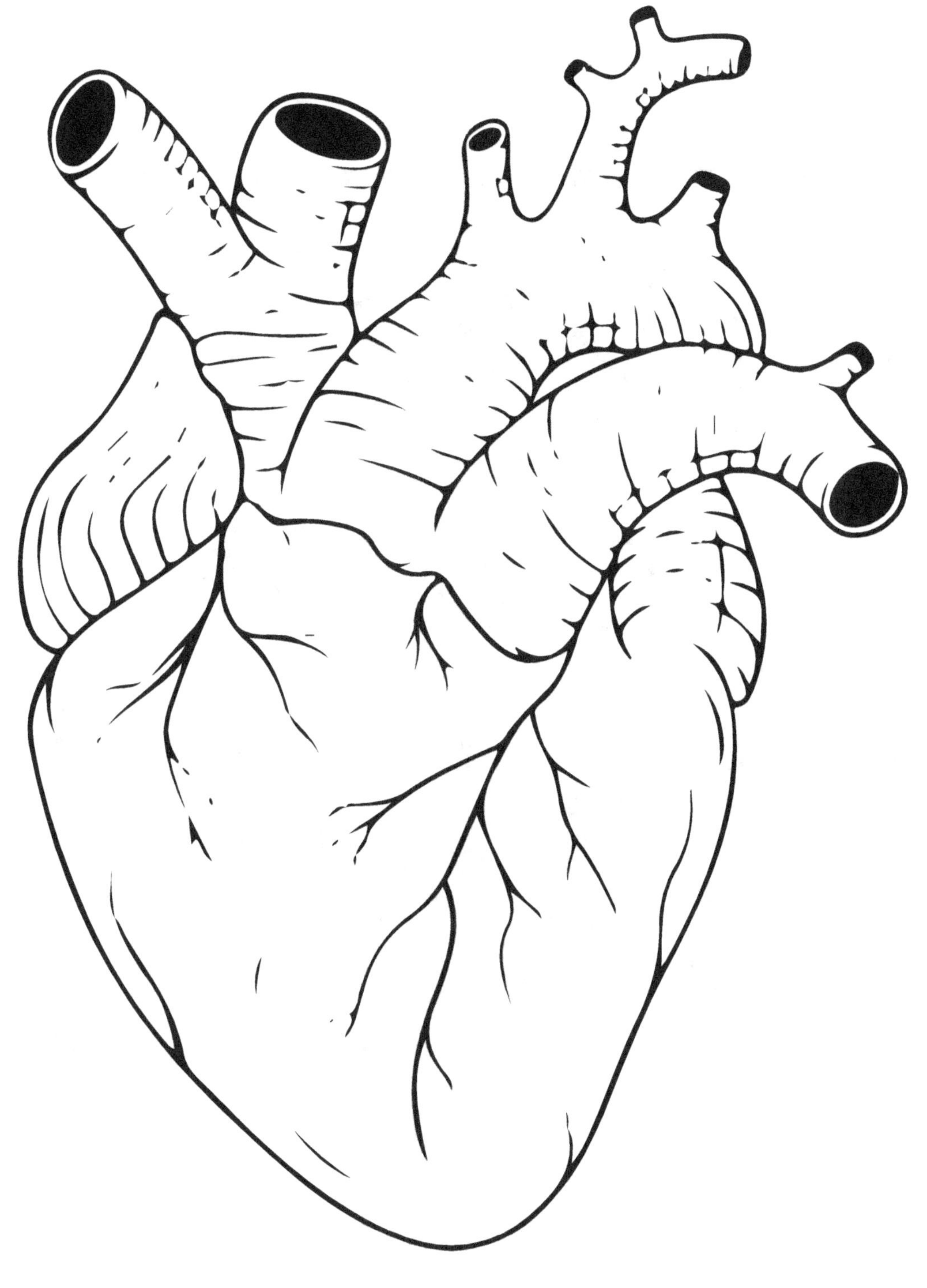

HEART

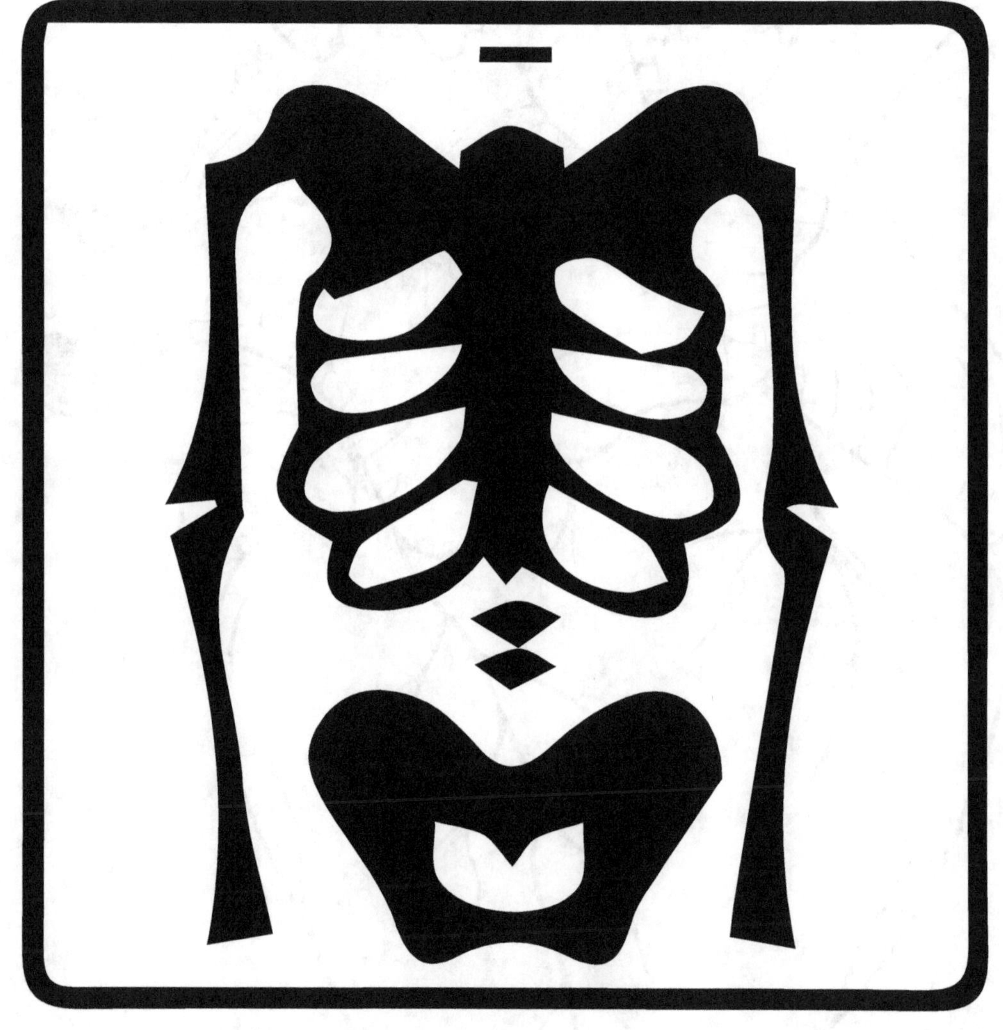

Radiology

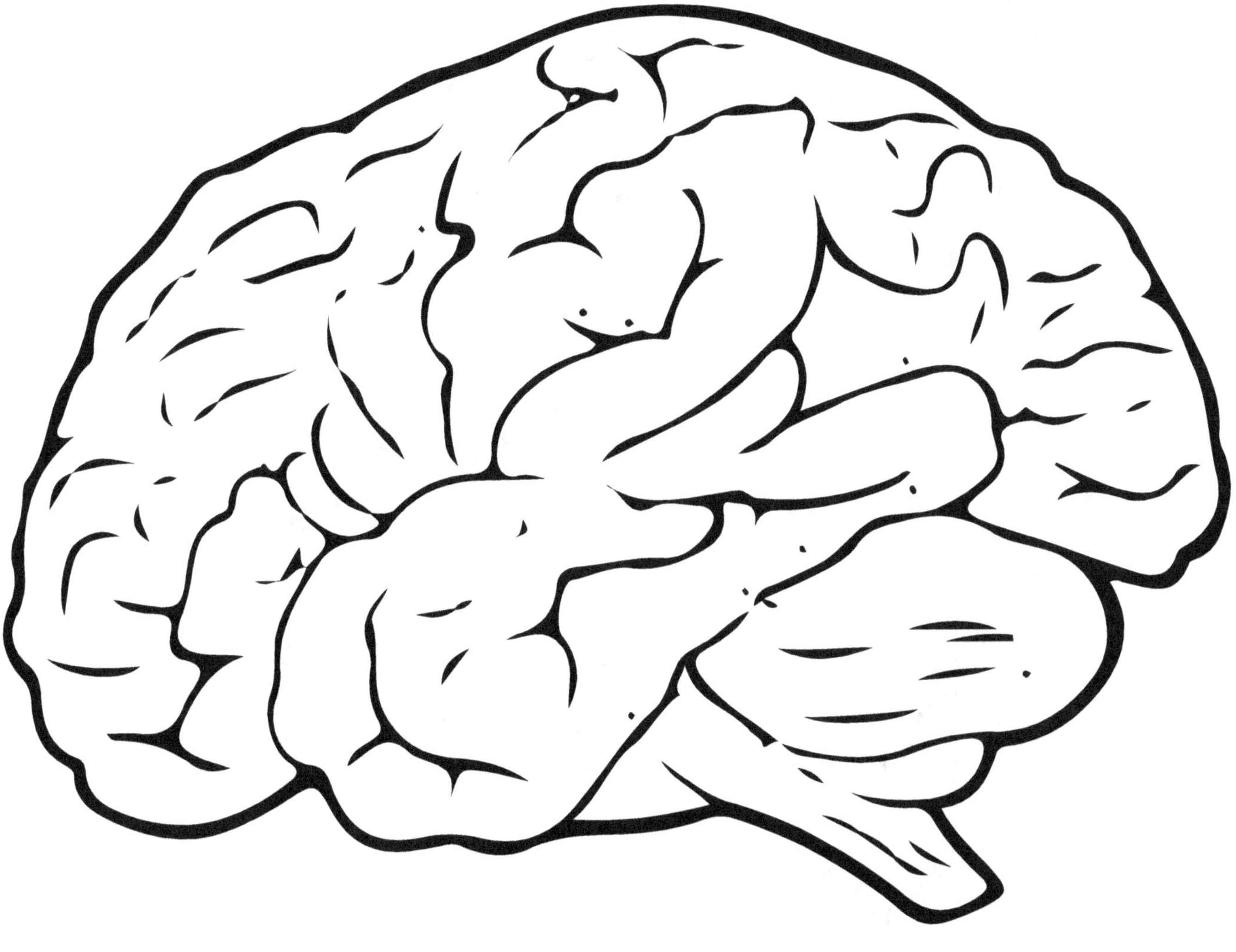

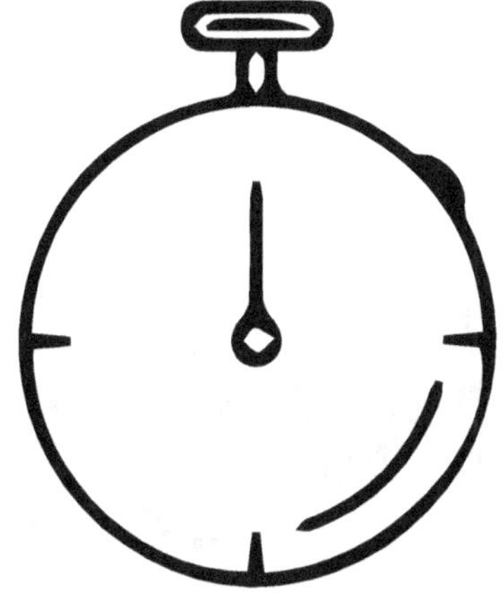

BRAIN

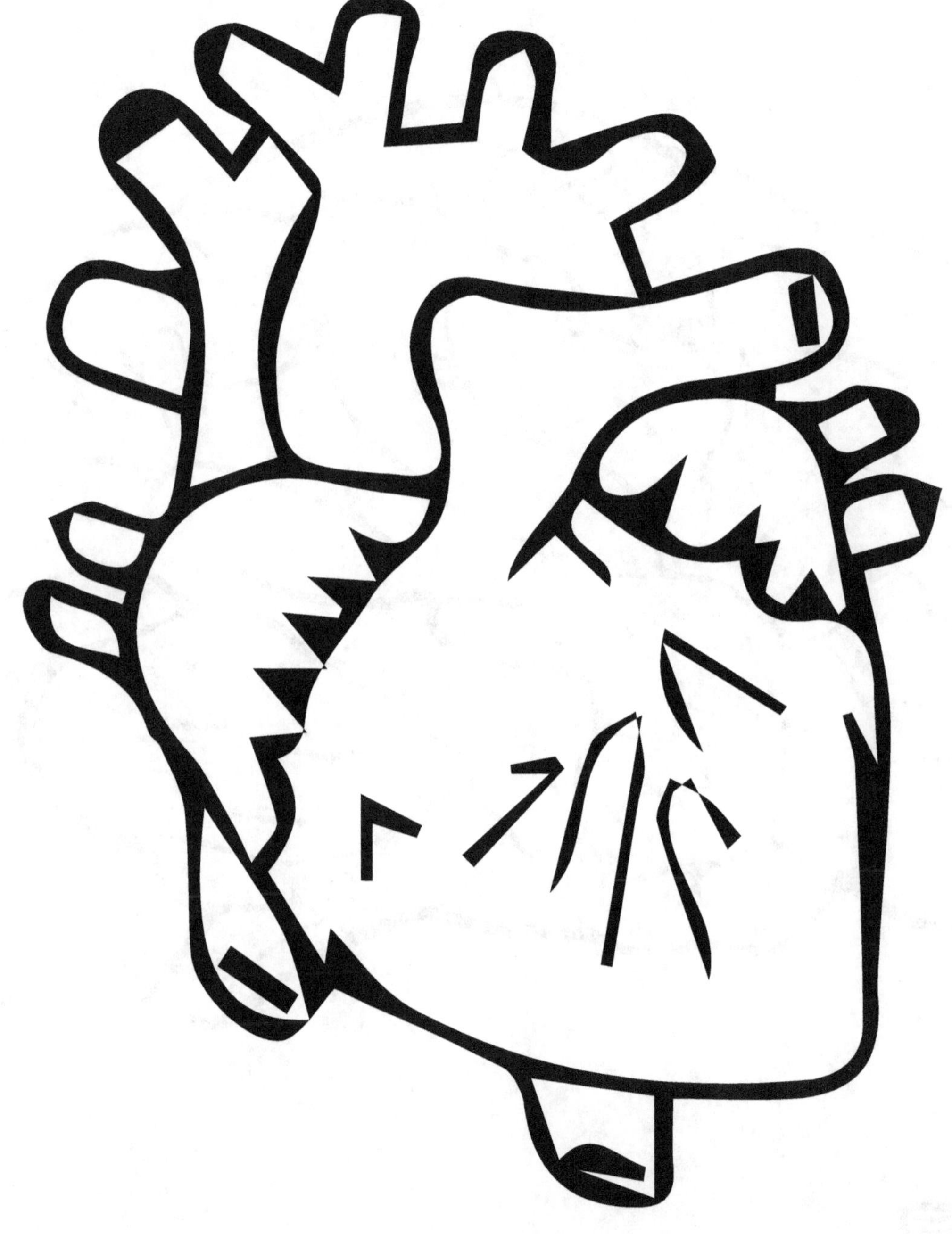

Pulmonology

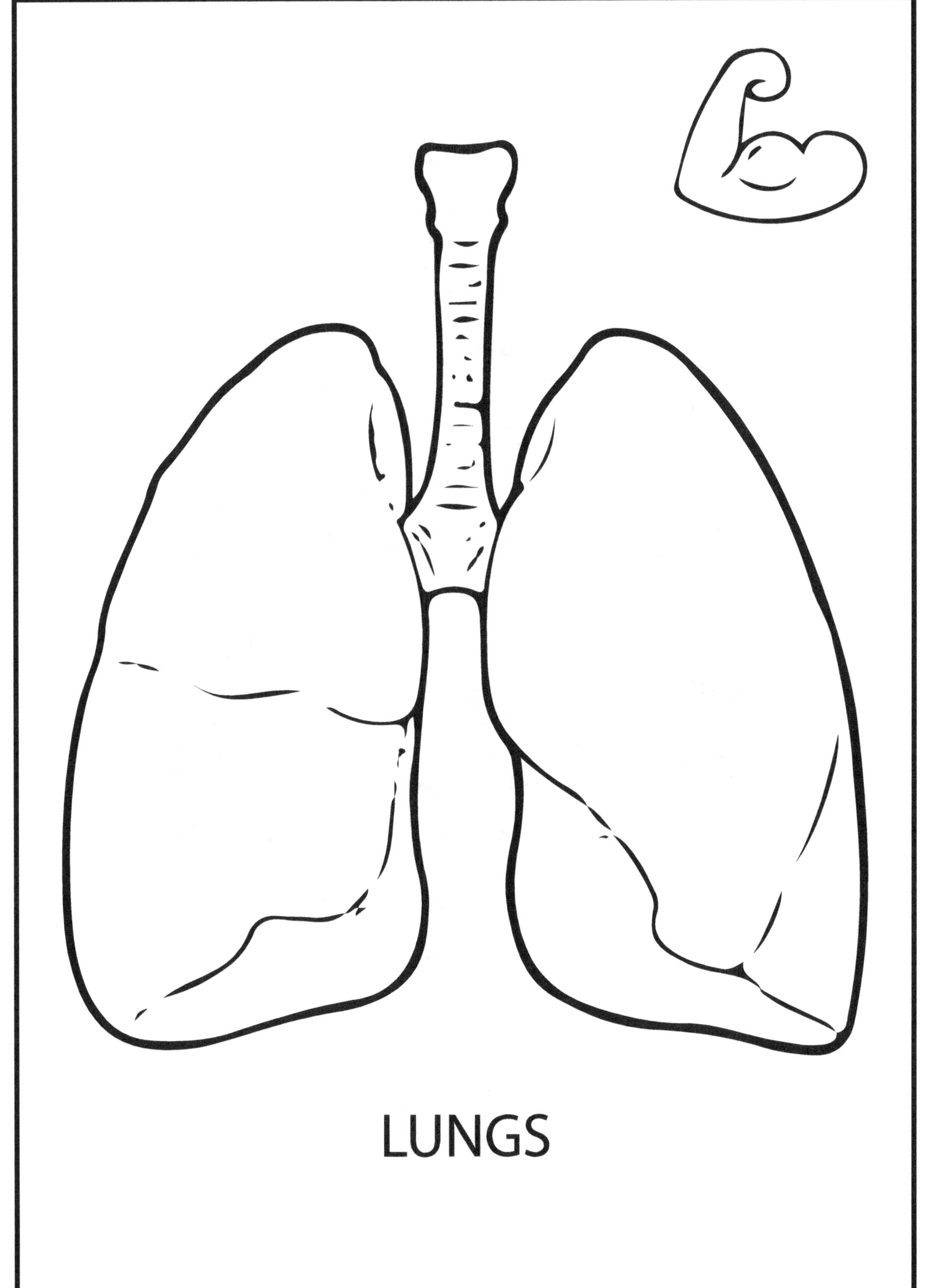

LUNGS

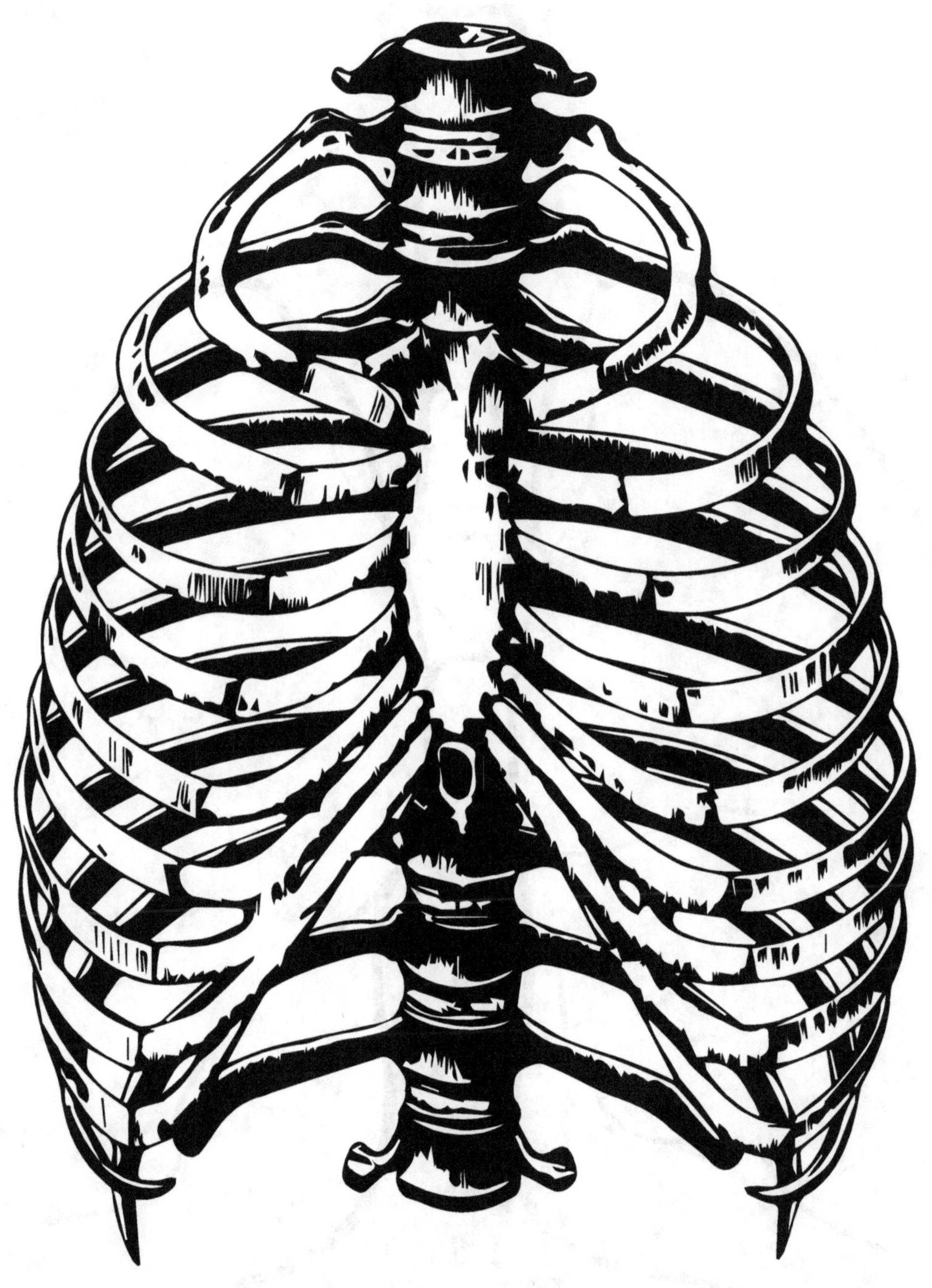

Anatomy Of Human Ribs

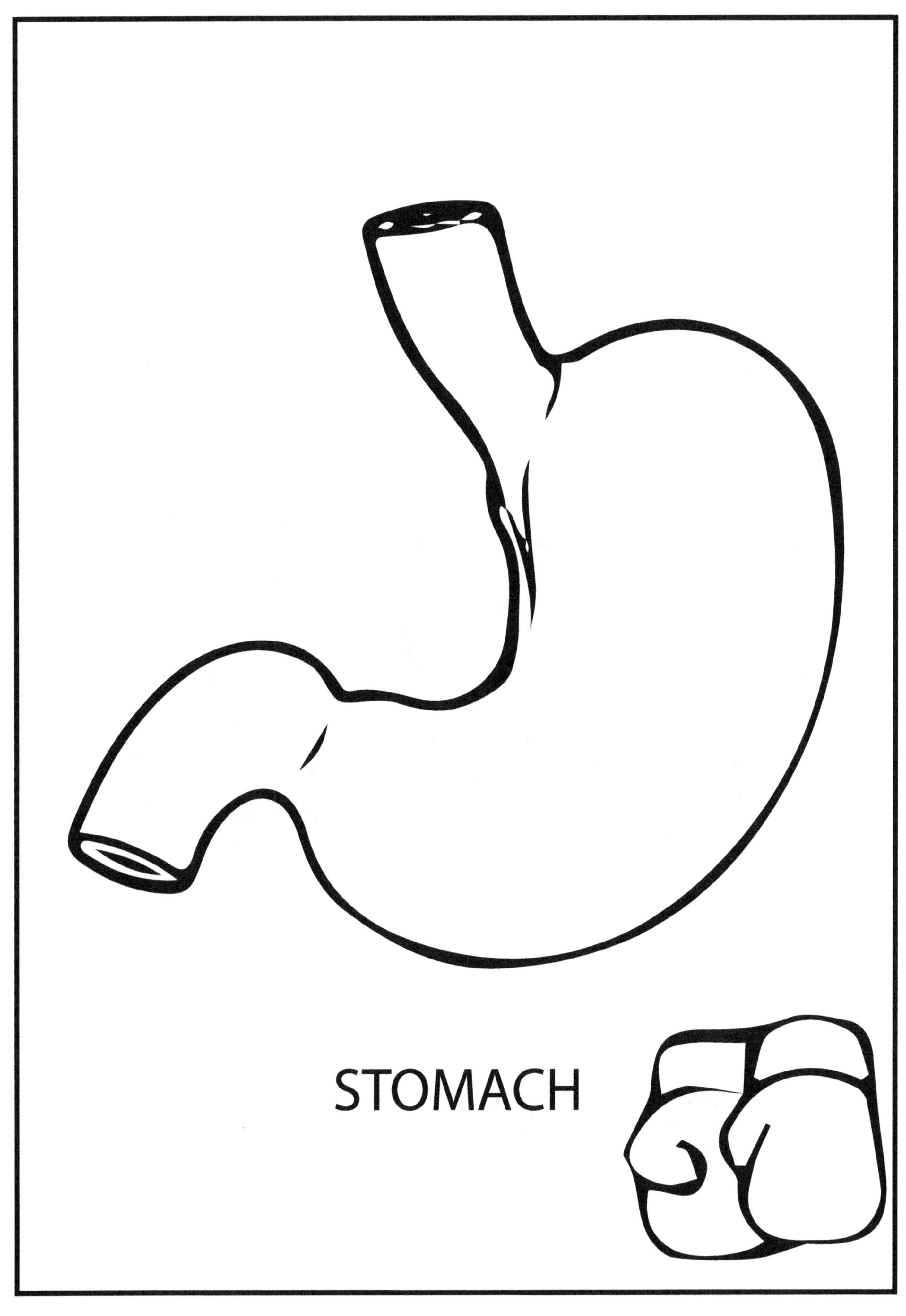

STOMACH

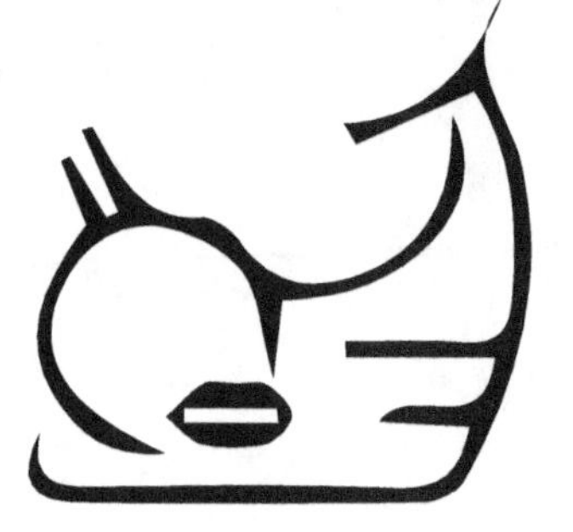

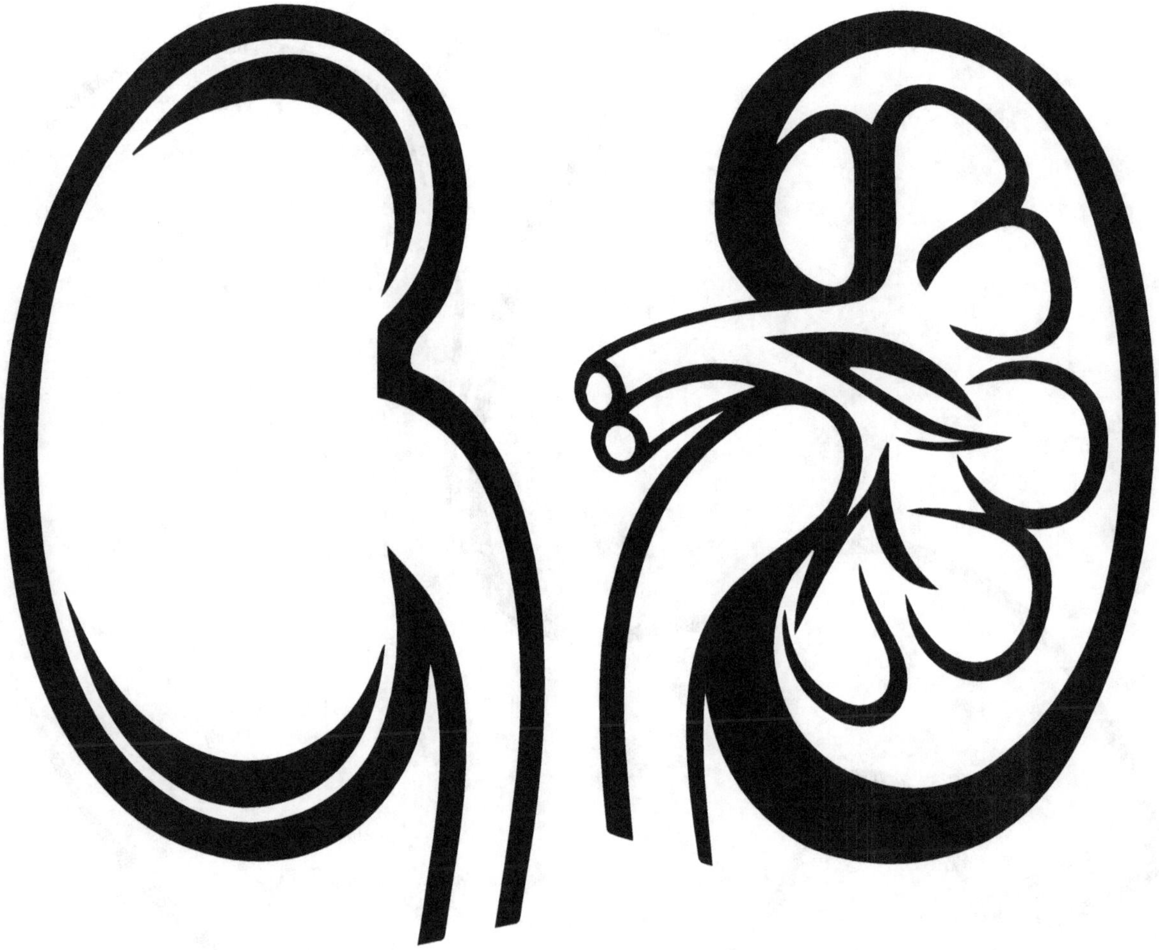

Human kidney

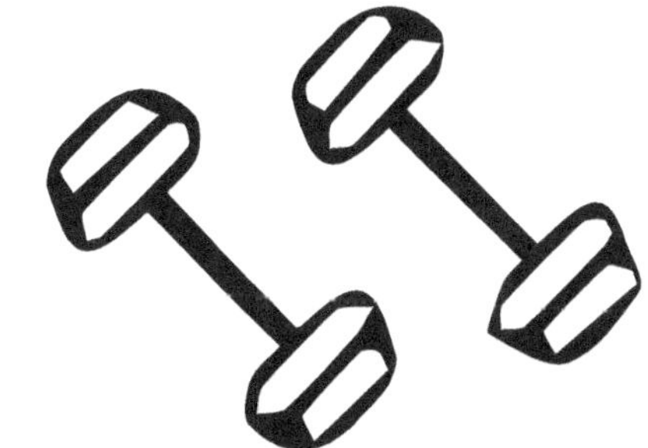

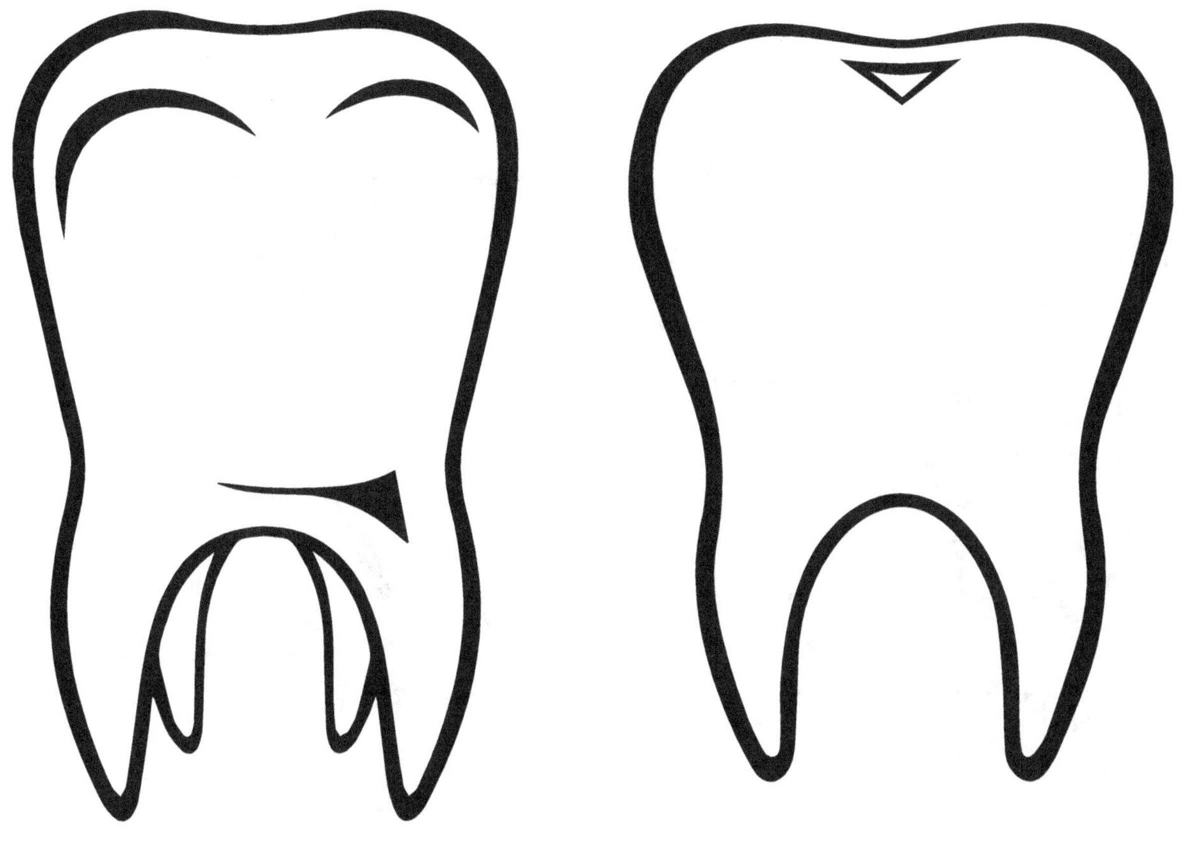

Tooth

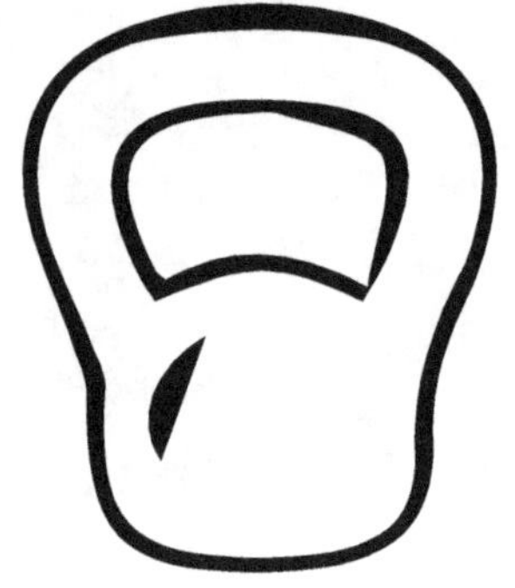

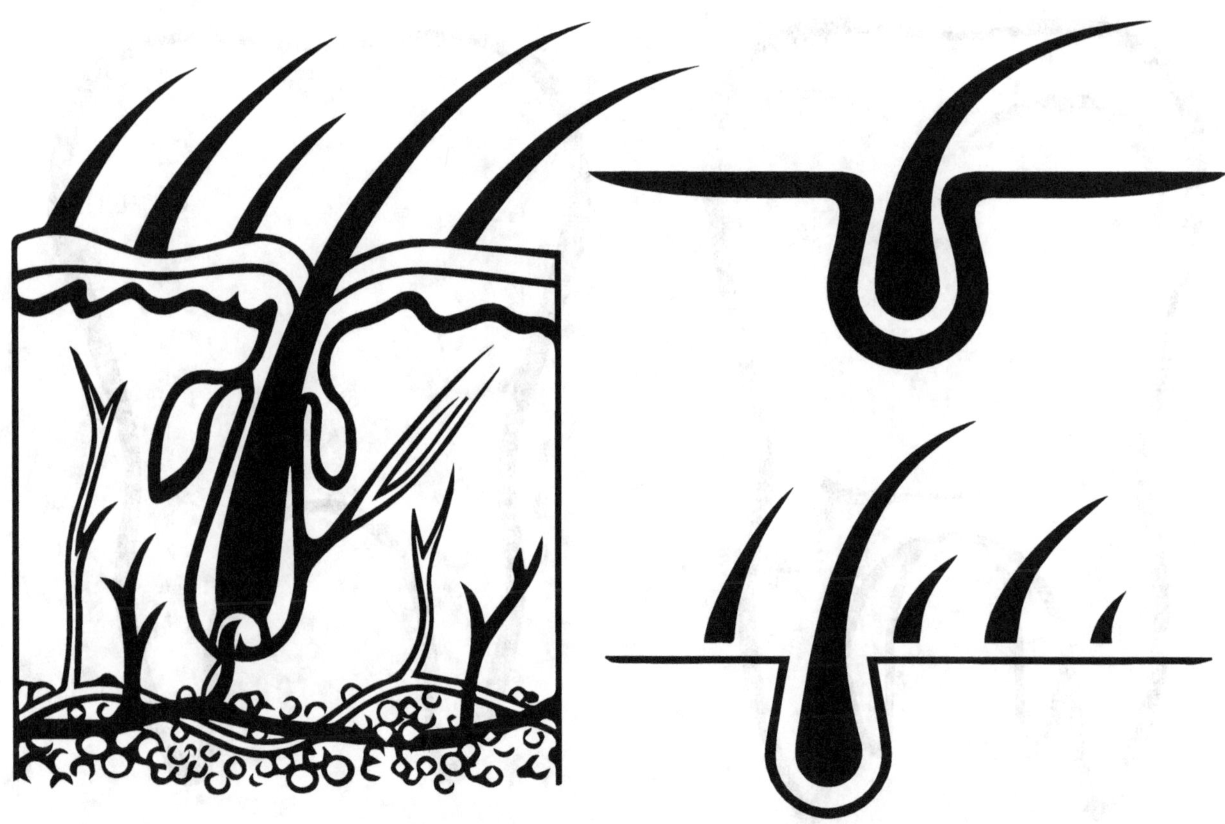

Human Hair

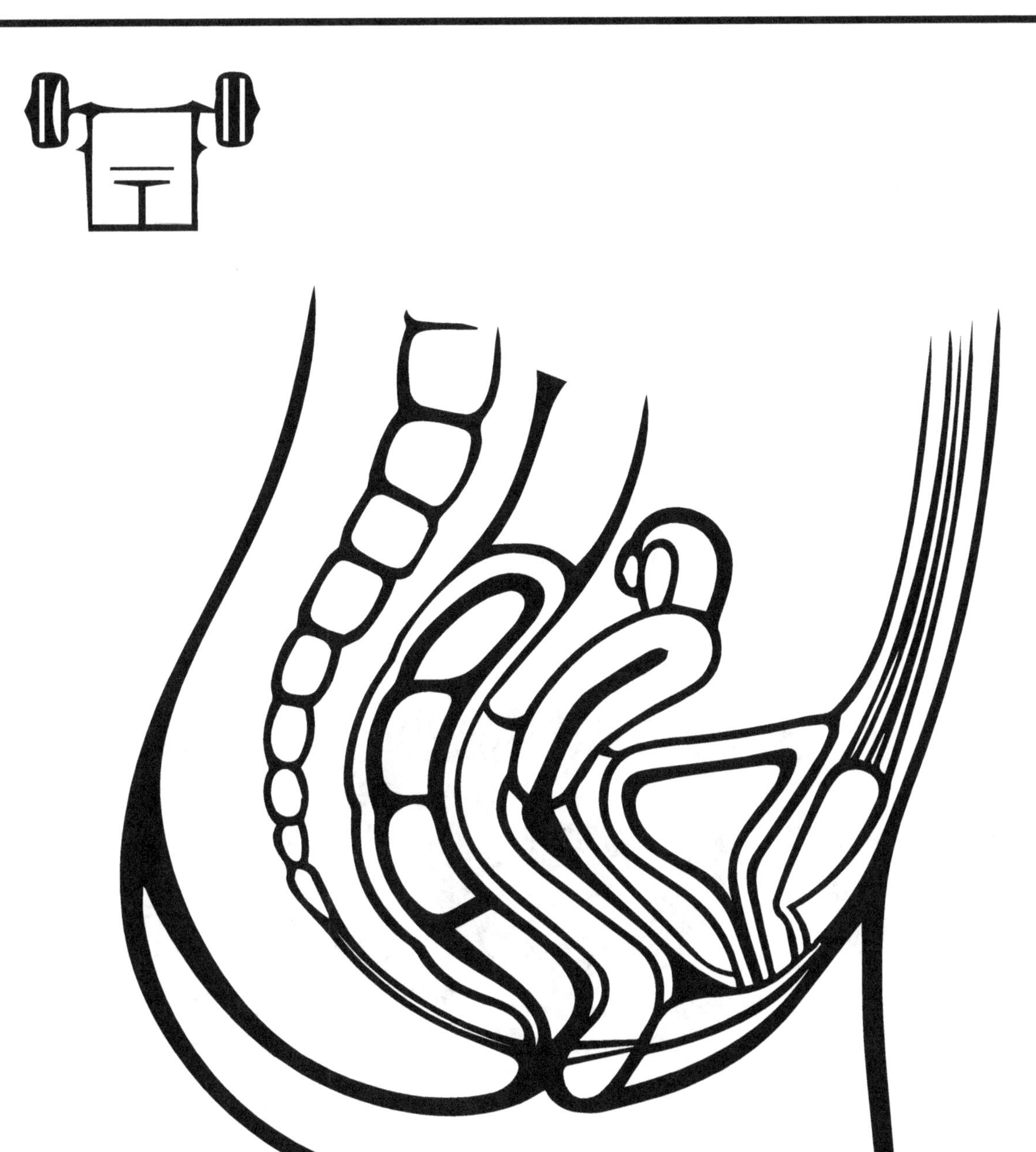

Femal urinary

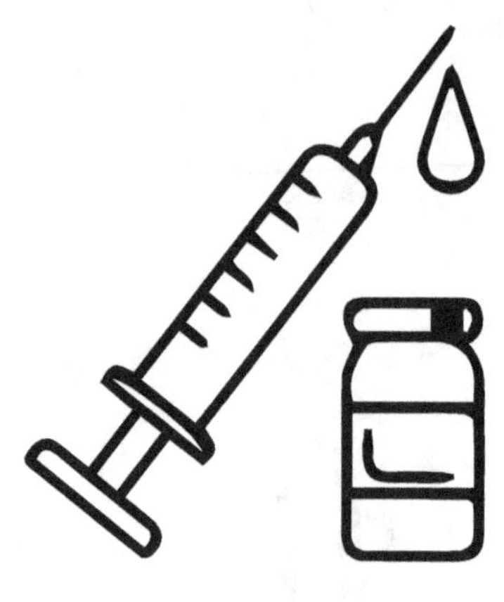

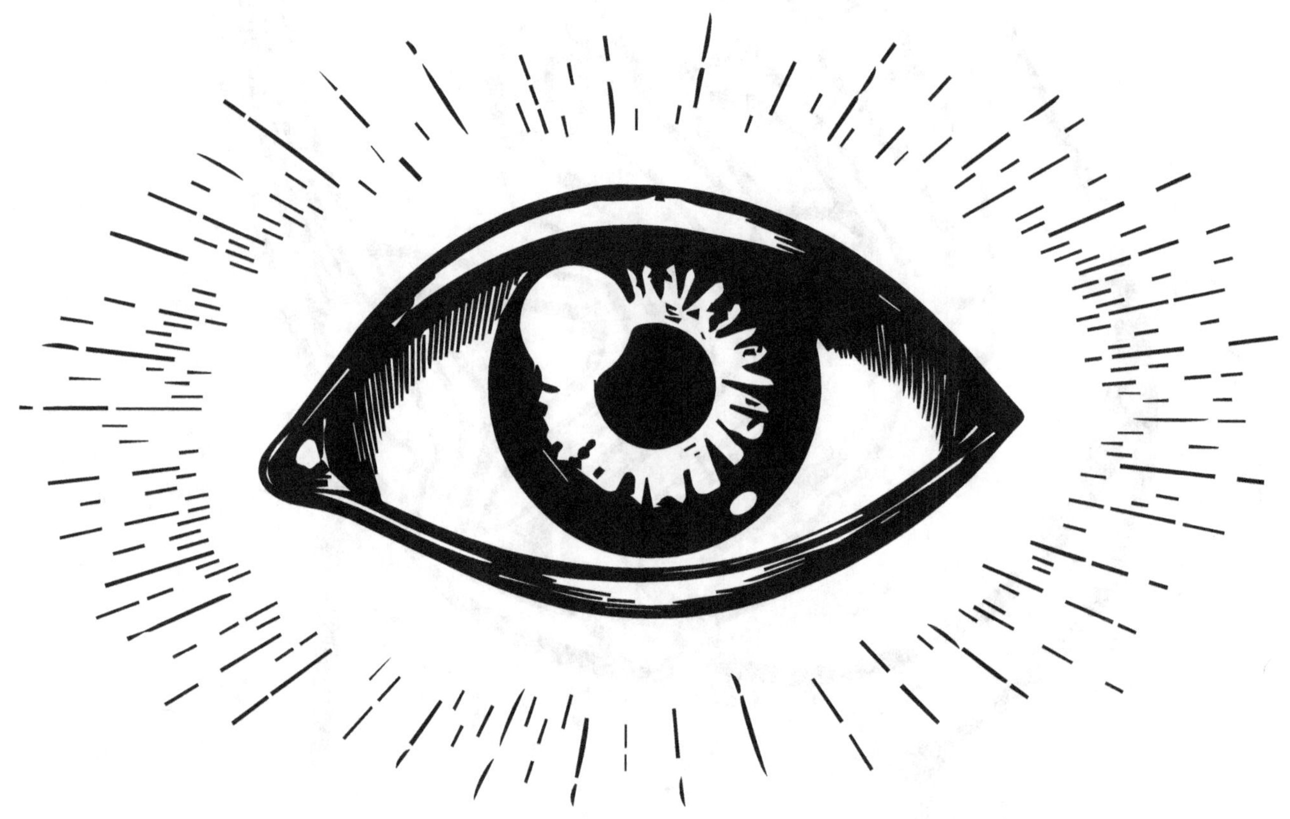

Pelvic bone anatomy

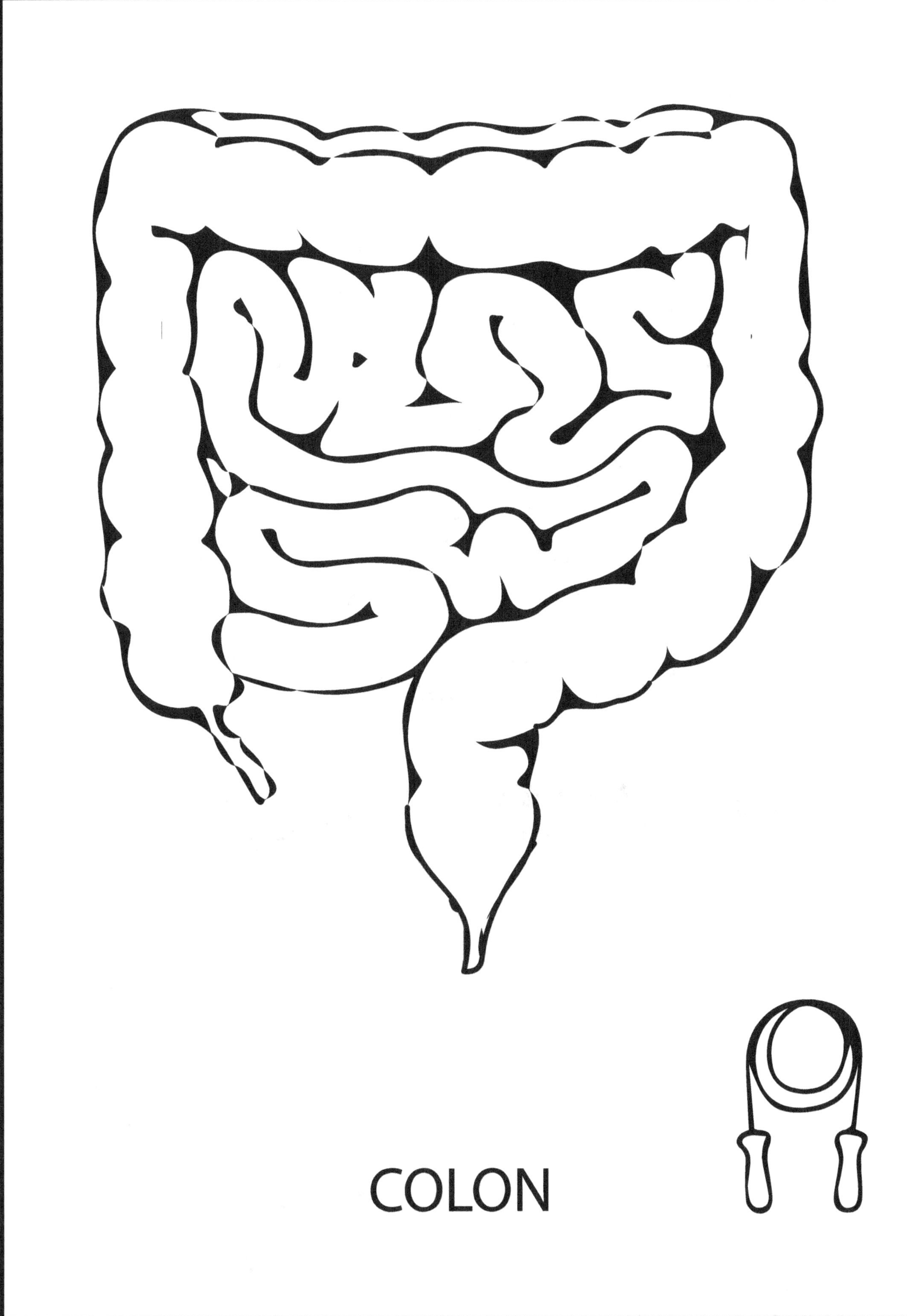

COLON

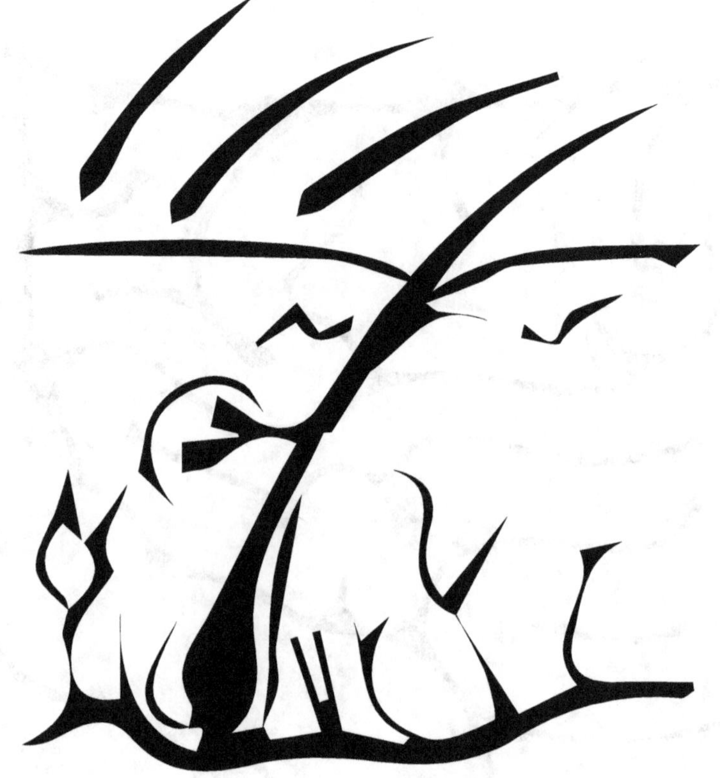

Dermatology

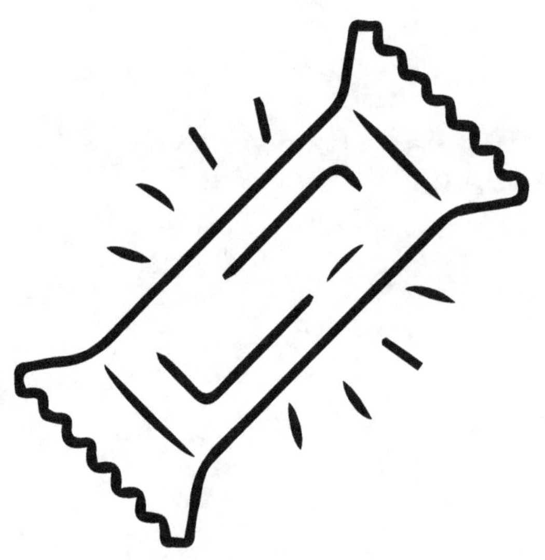

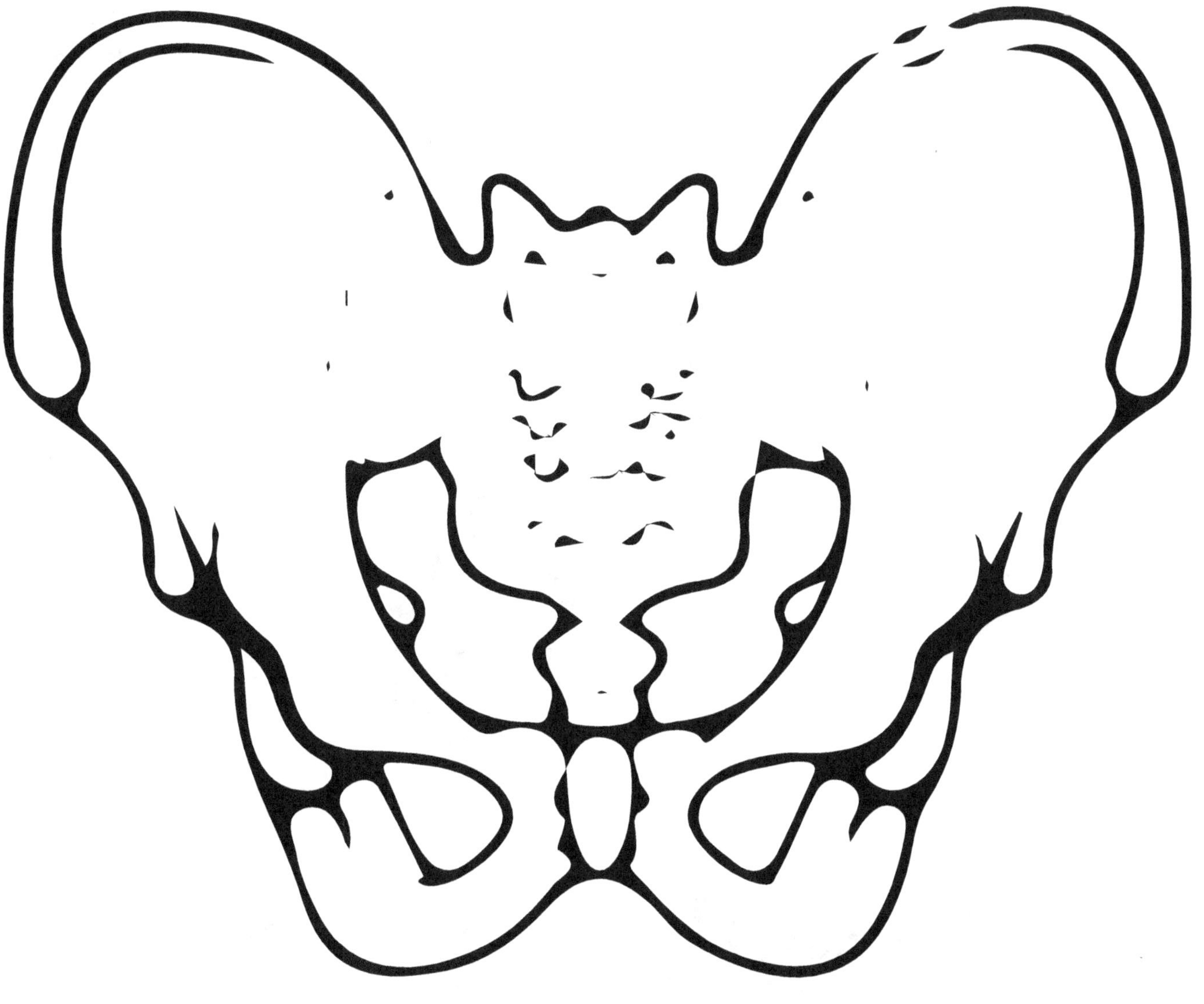

PELVIS

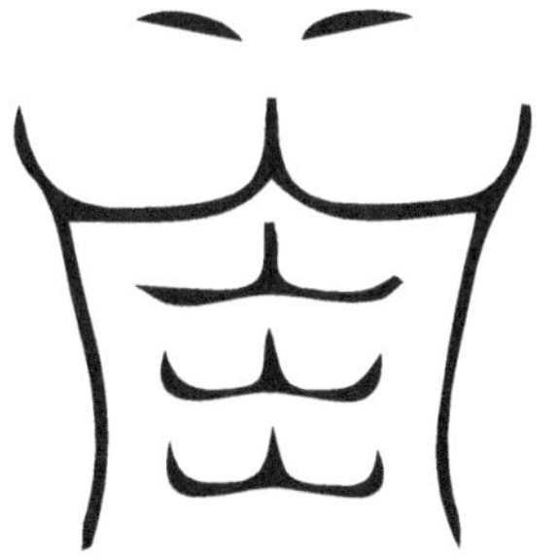

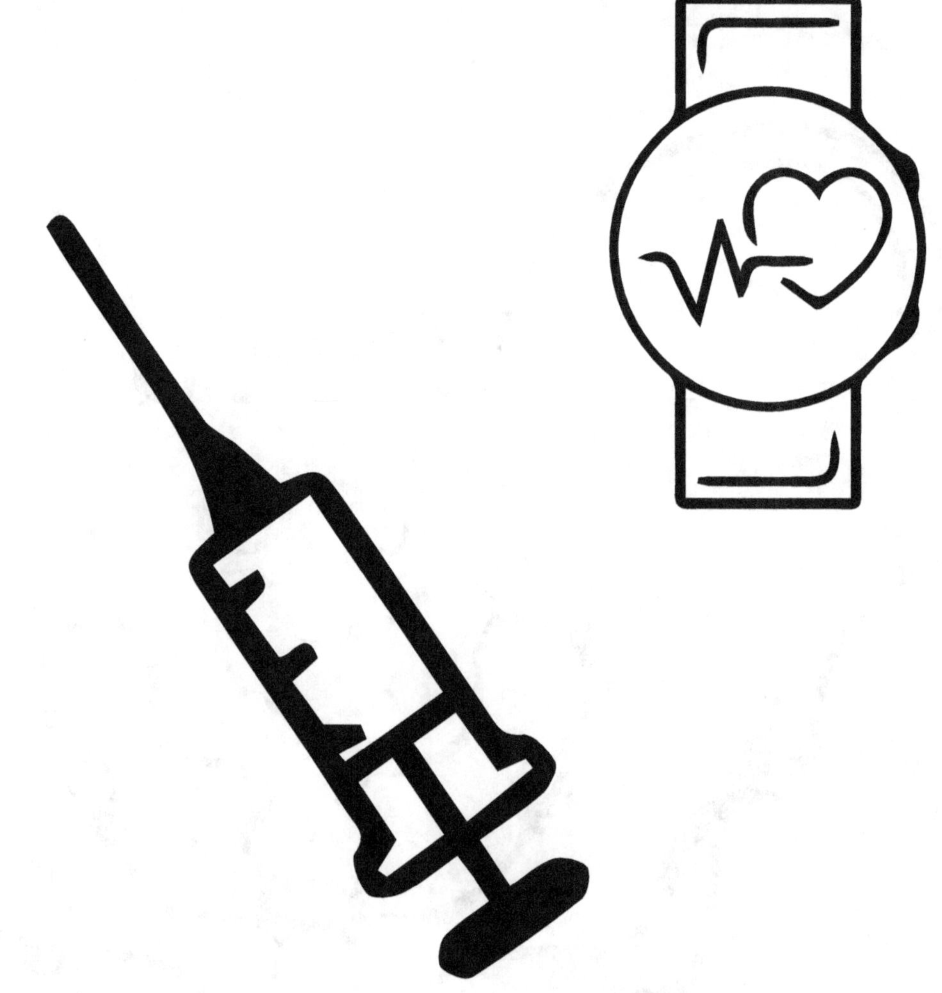

Anesthesiology

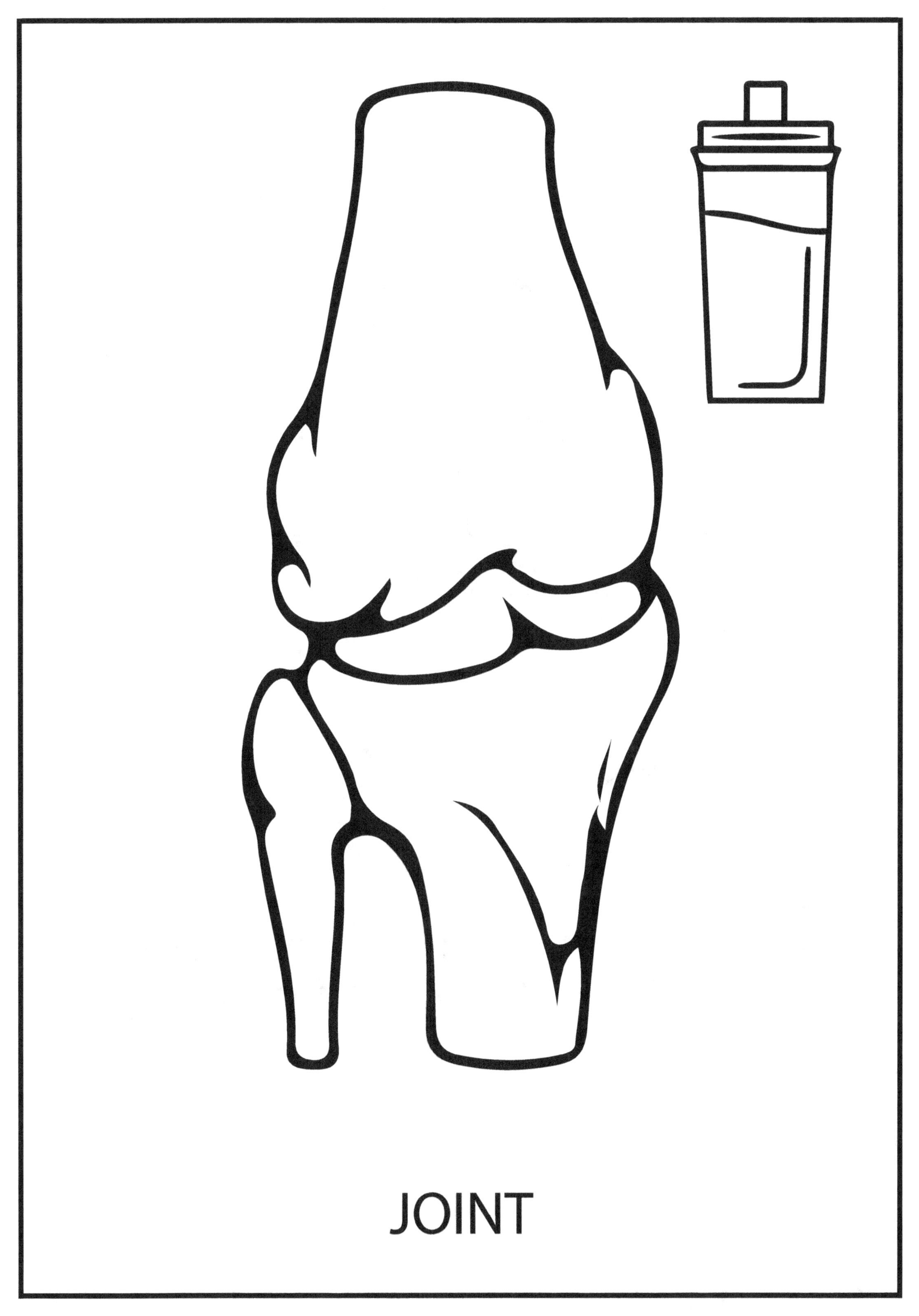

JOINT

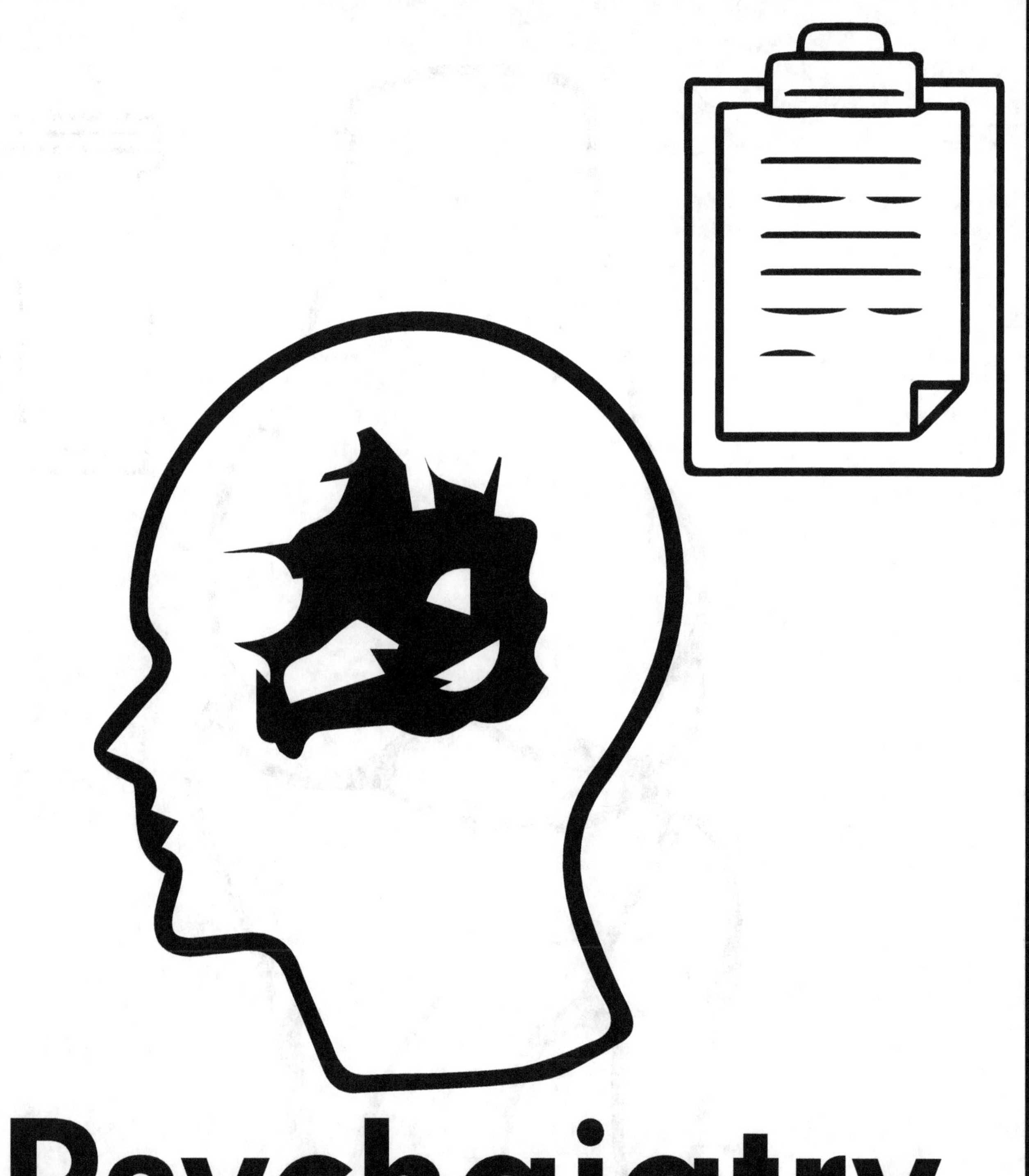

Psychaiatry

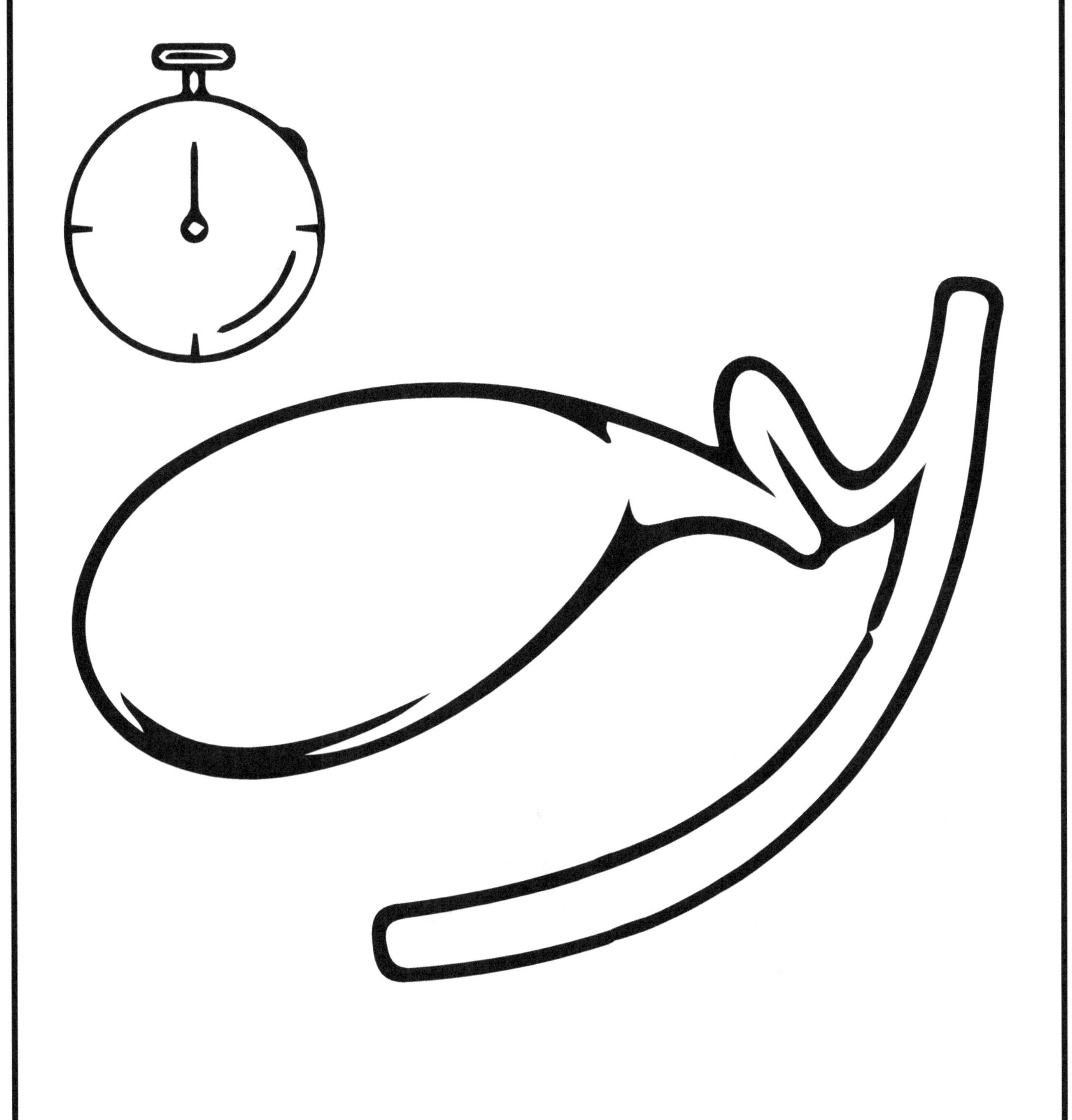

GALLABLADDER

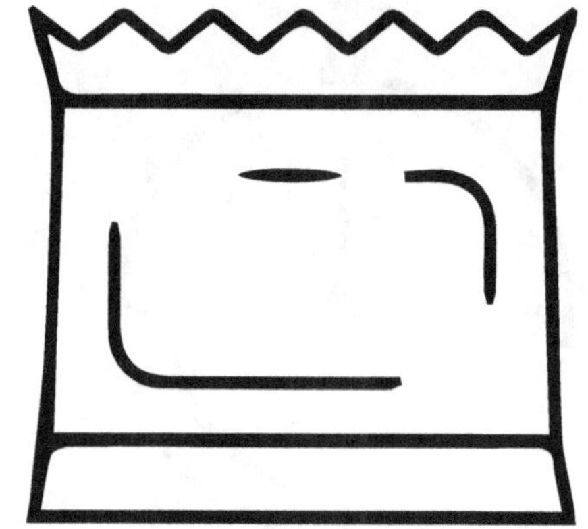

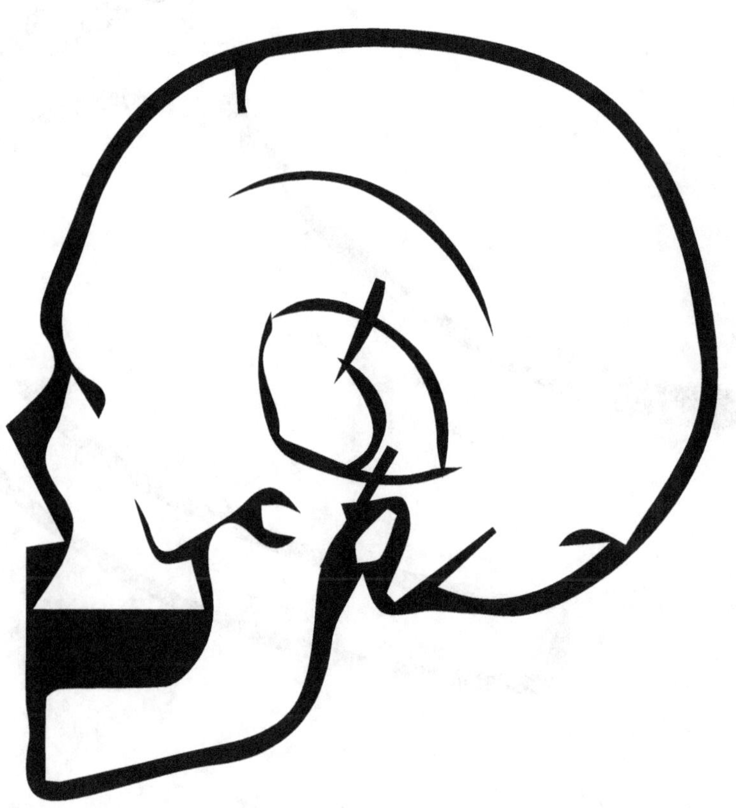

Traumatology

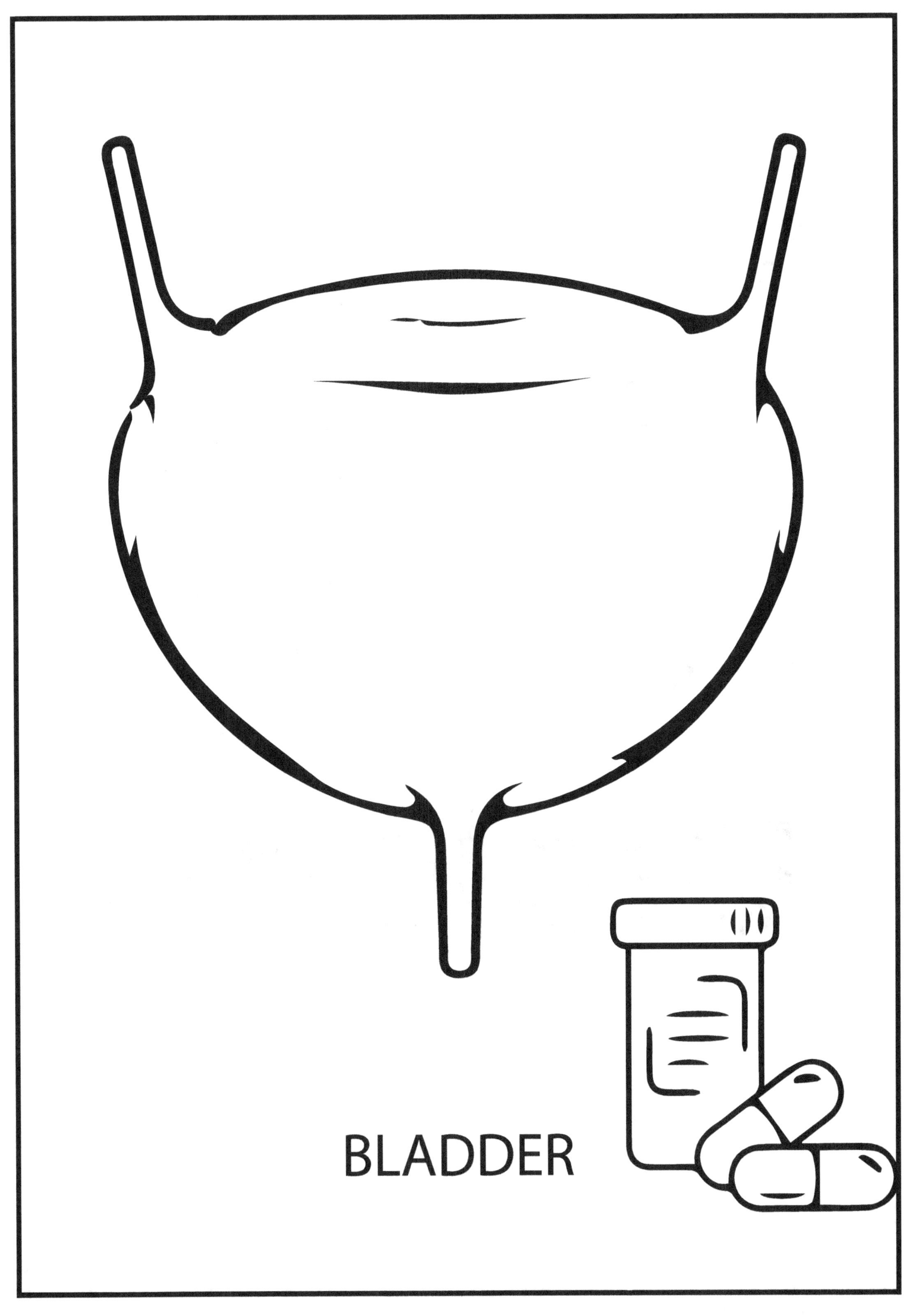
BLADDER

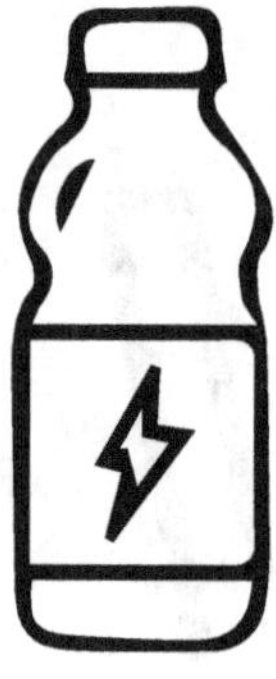

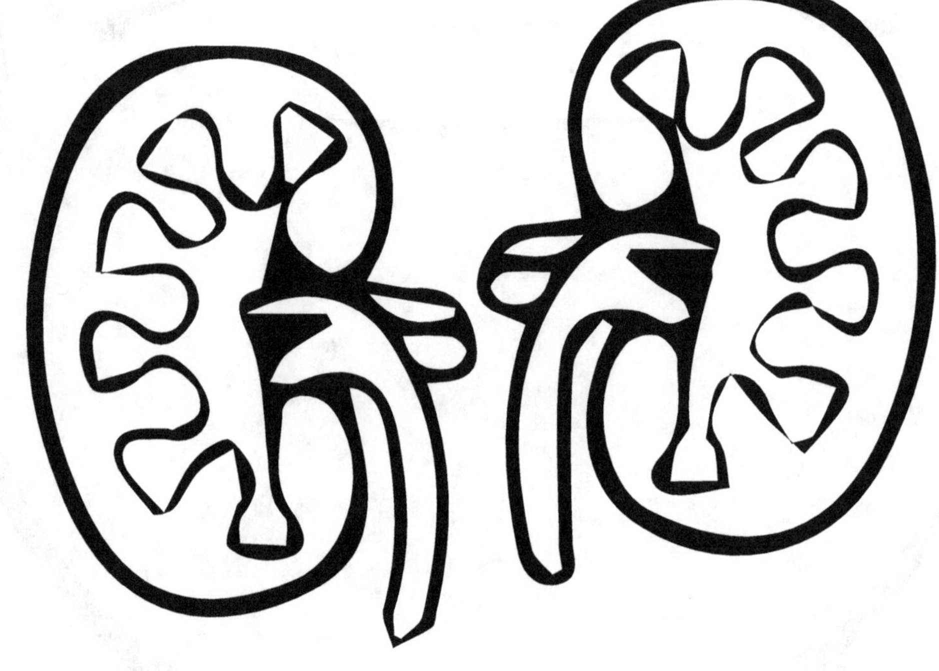

Urology

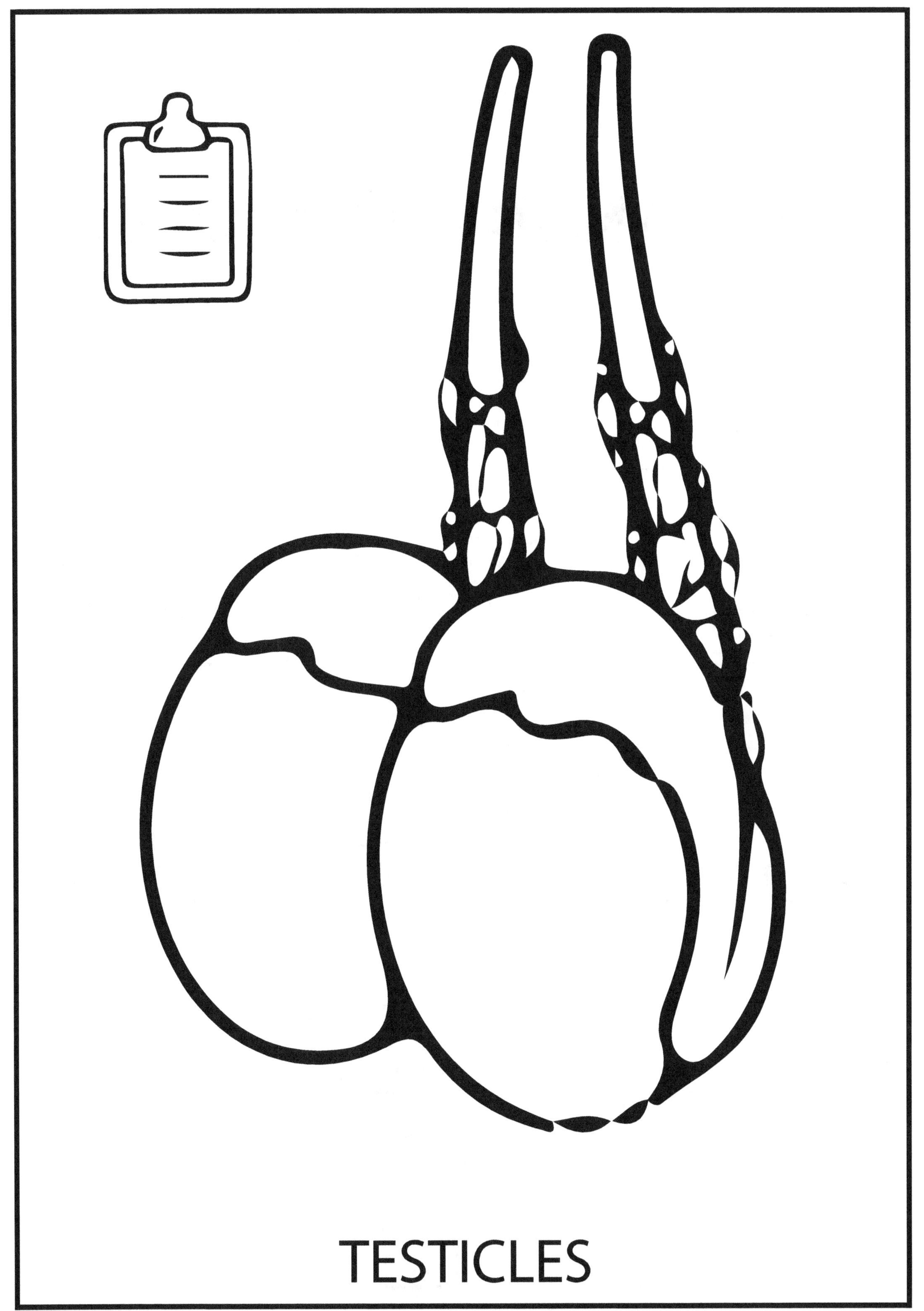

TESTICLES

PREGNANT ANATOMY

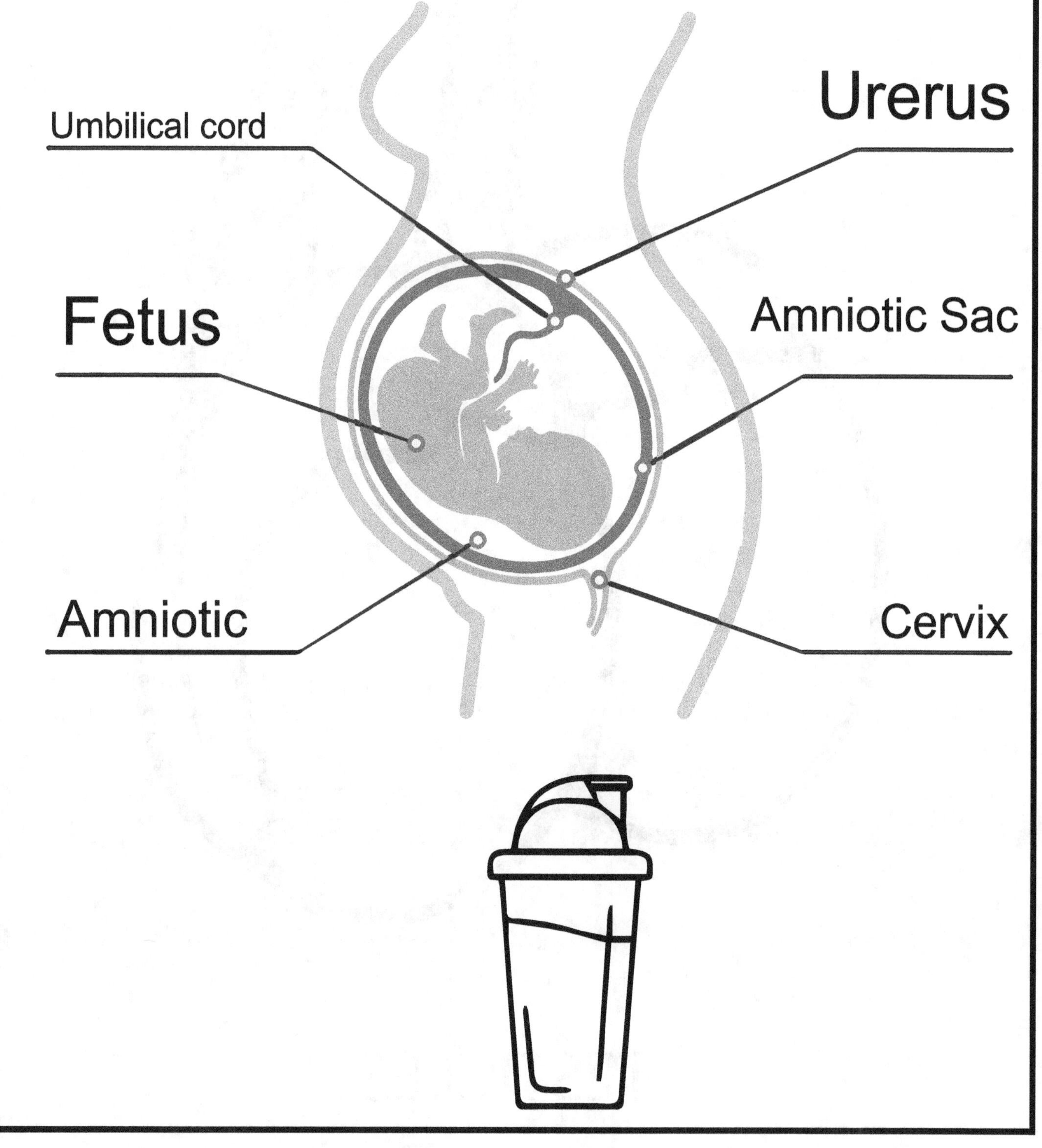

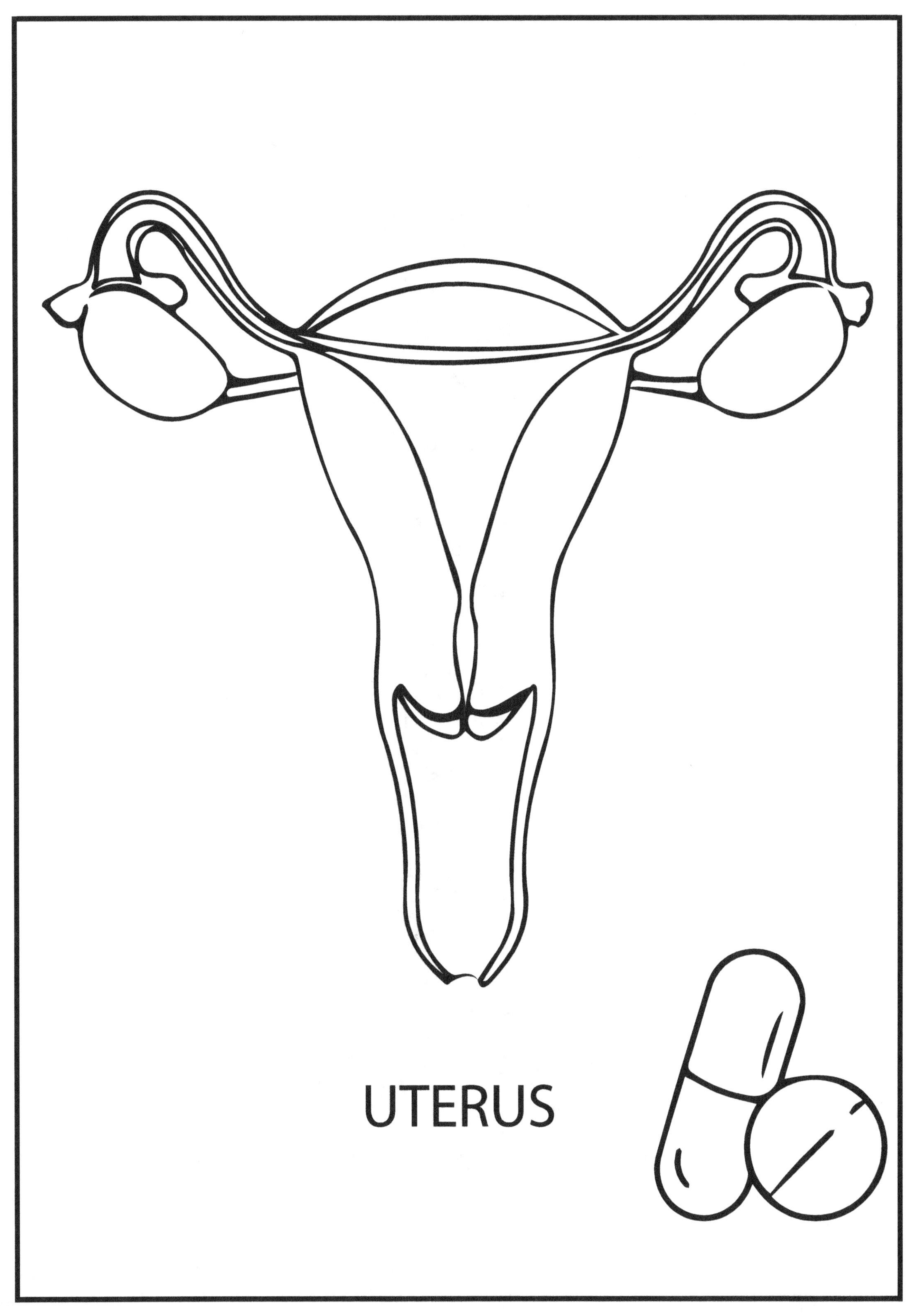

UTERUS

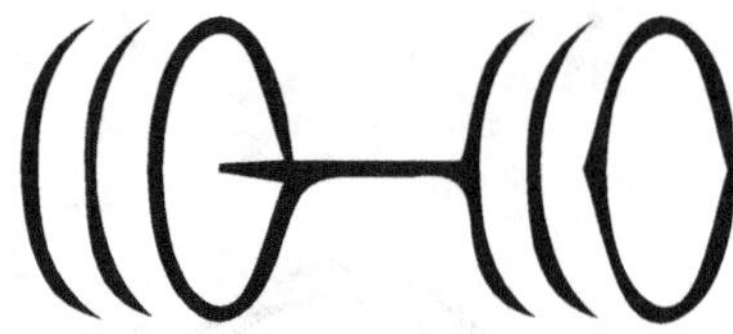

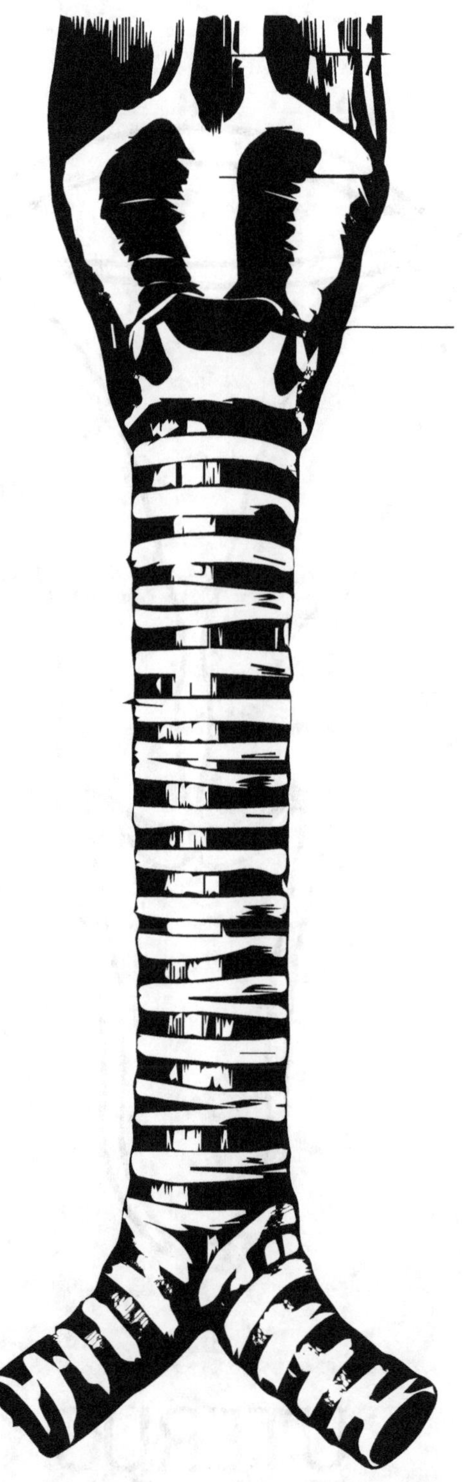

Anatomy of the Trachea and larynx

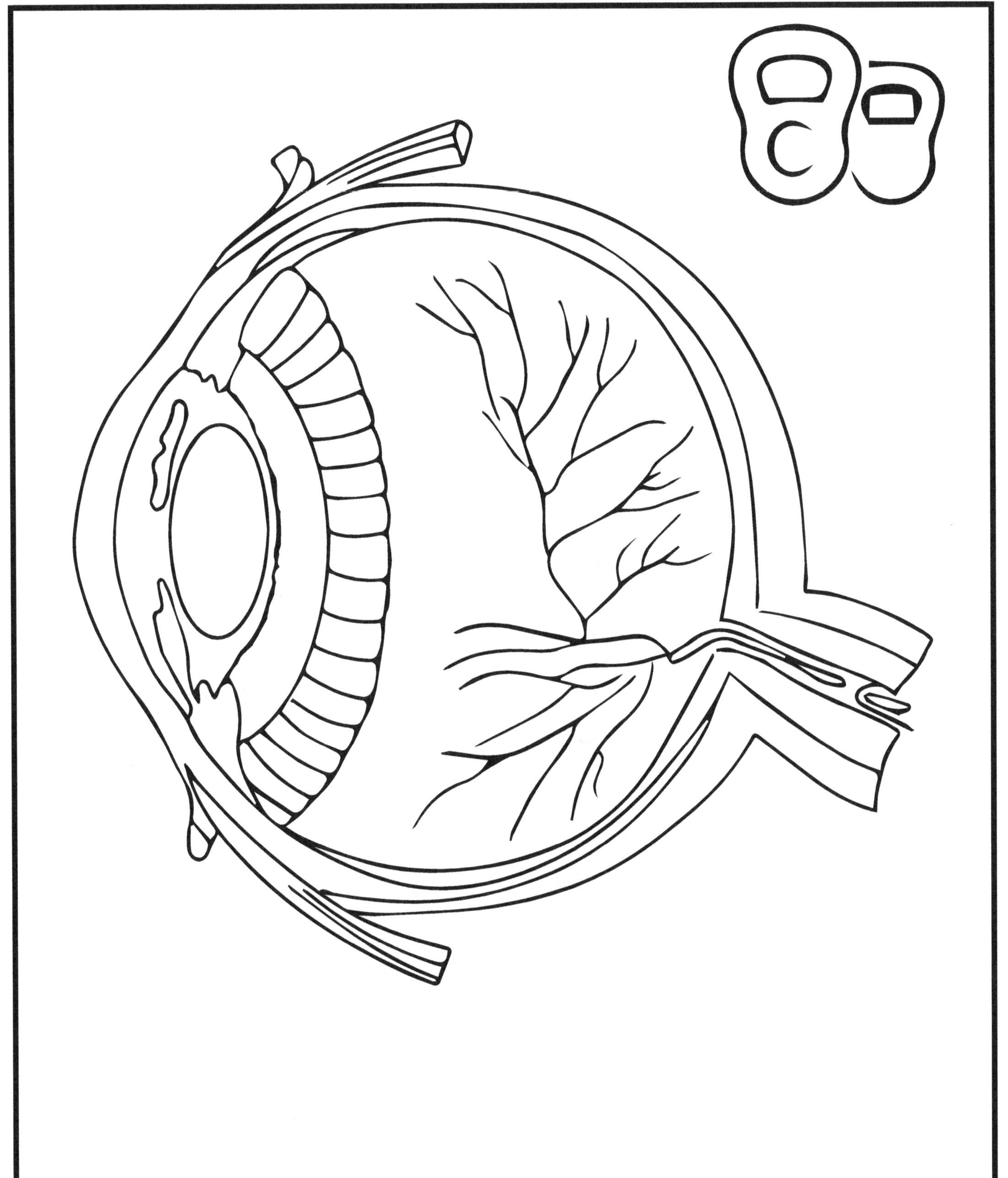

HUMAN EYE STRUCTURE

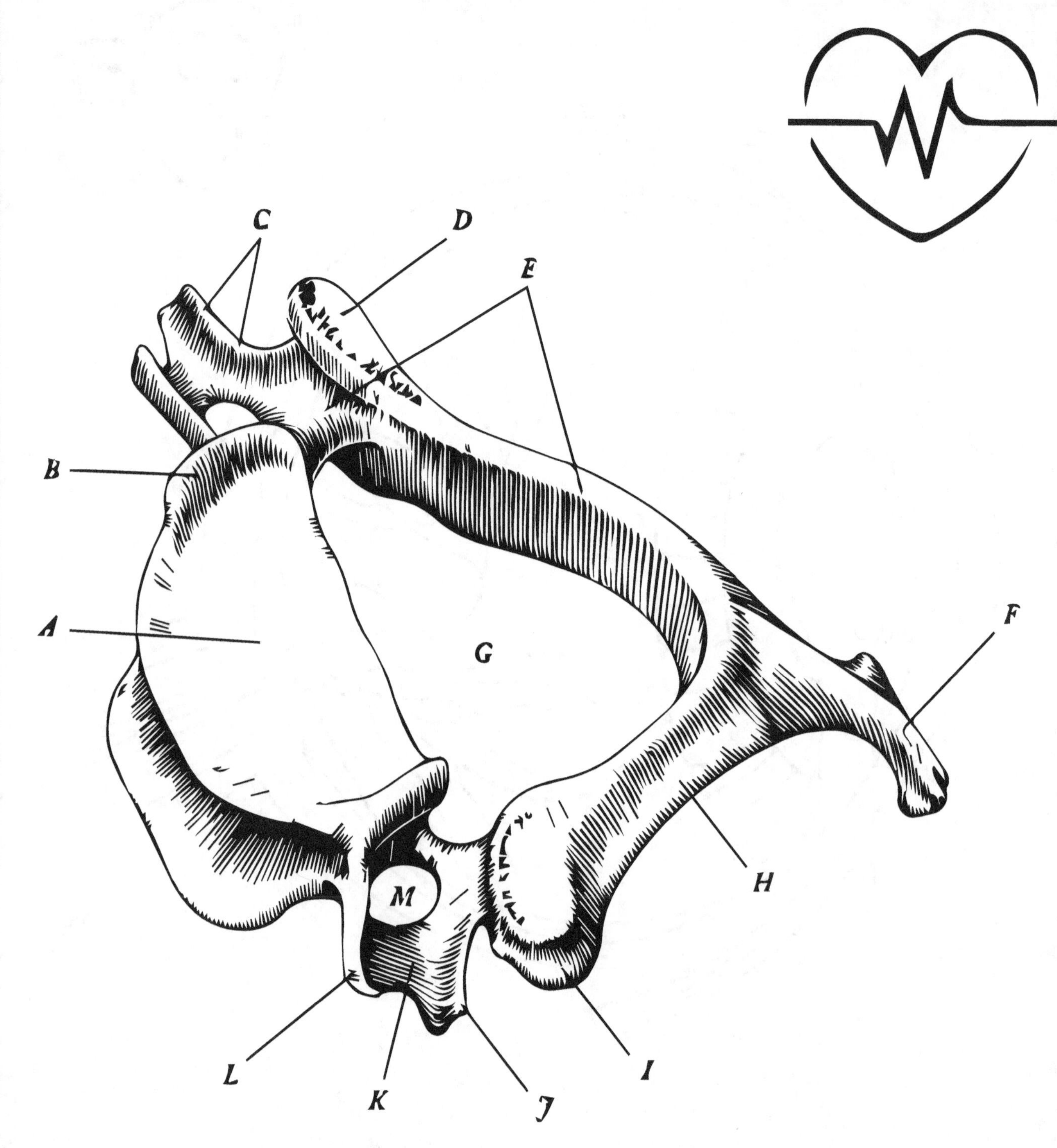

Cervical vertebra

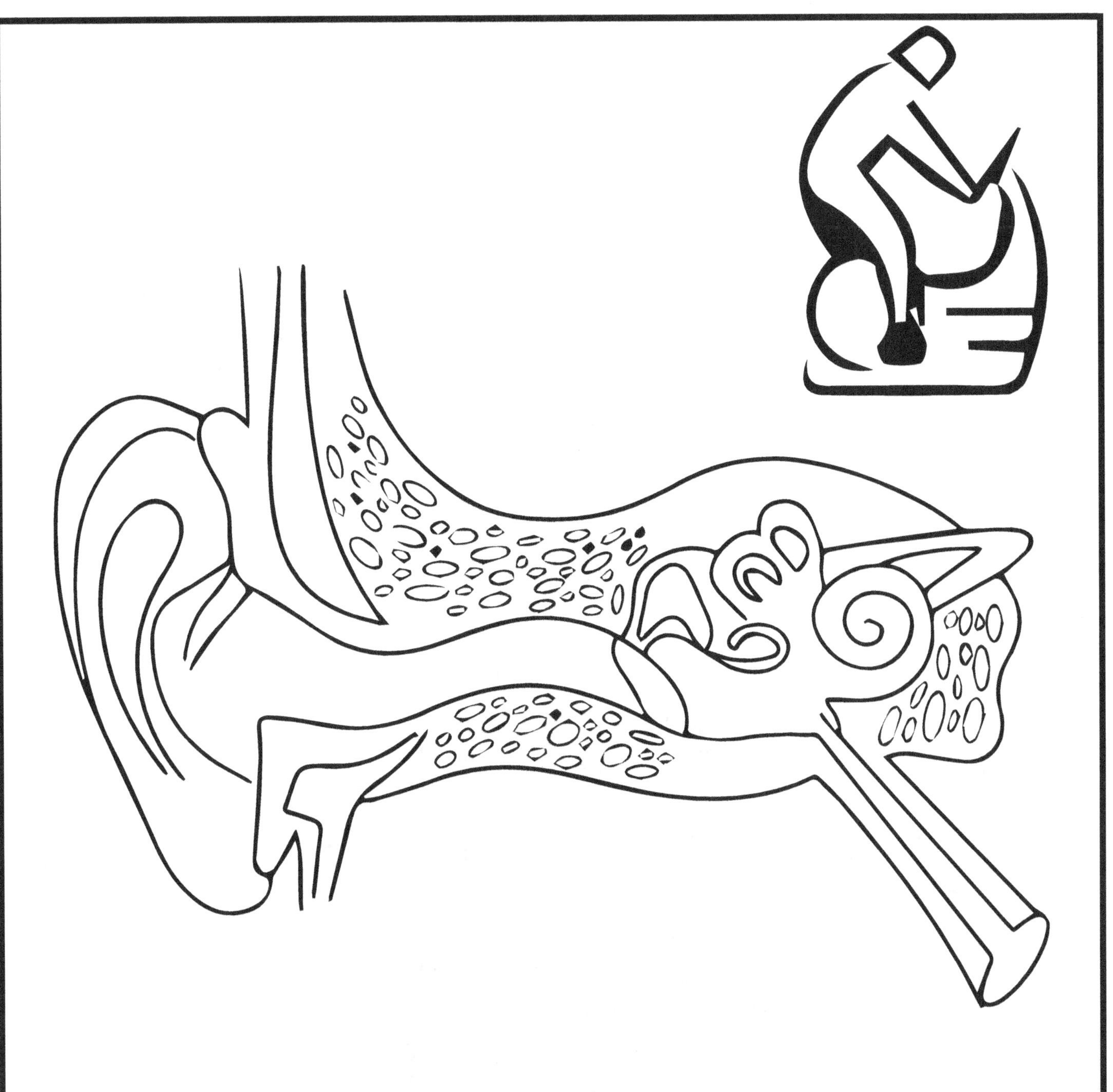

HUMAN EAR STRUCTURE

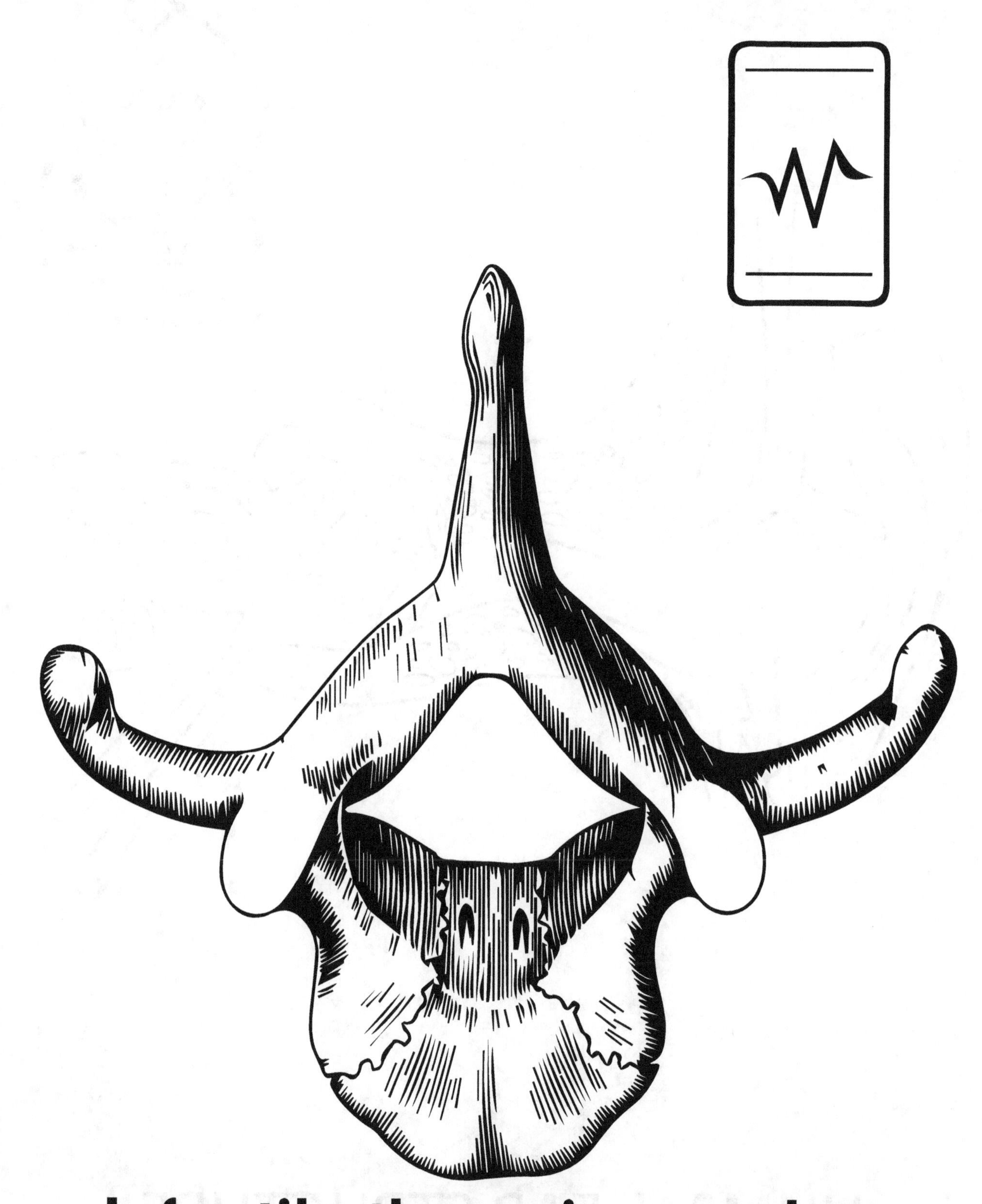

Infantile thoracic vertebra

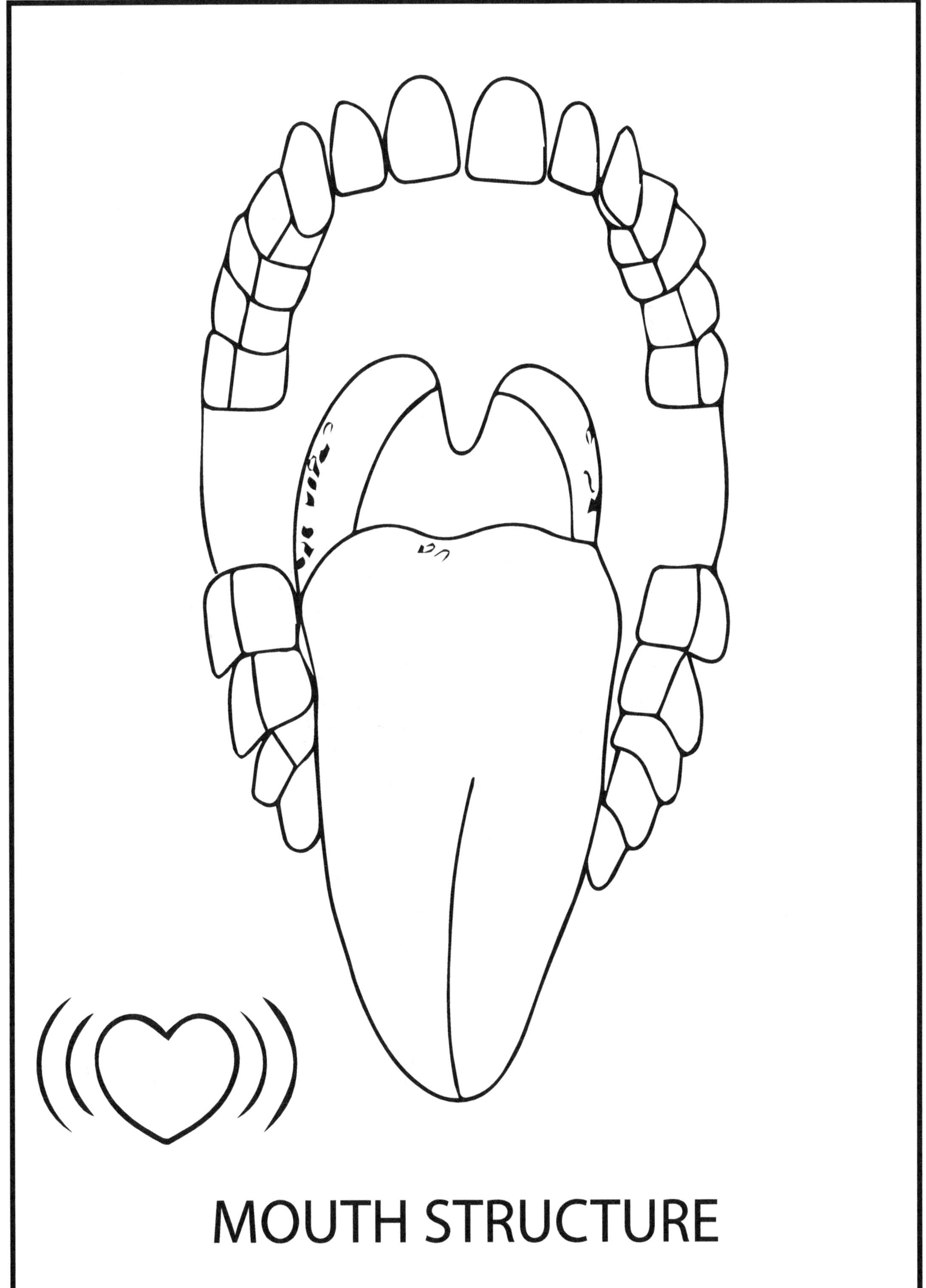

MOUTH STRUCTURE

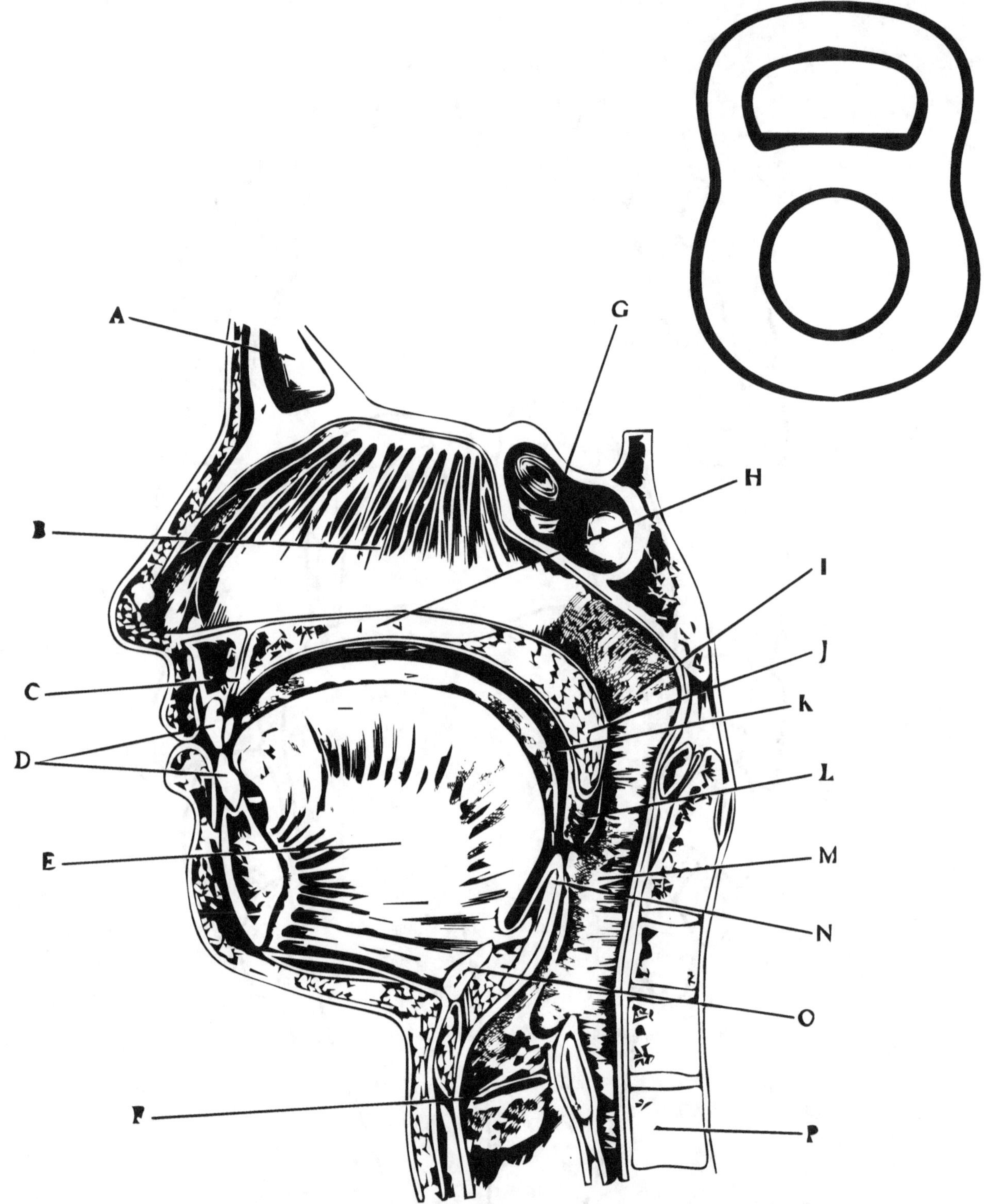

Antique engraving human oral cavity

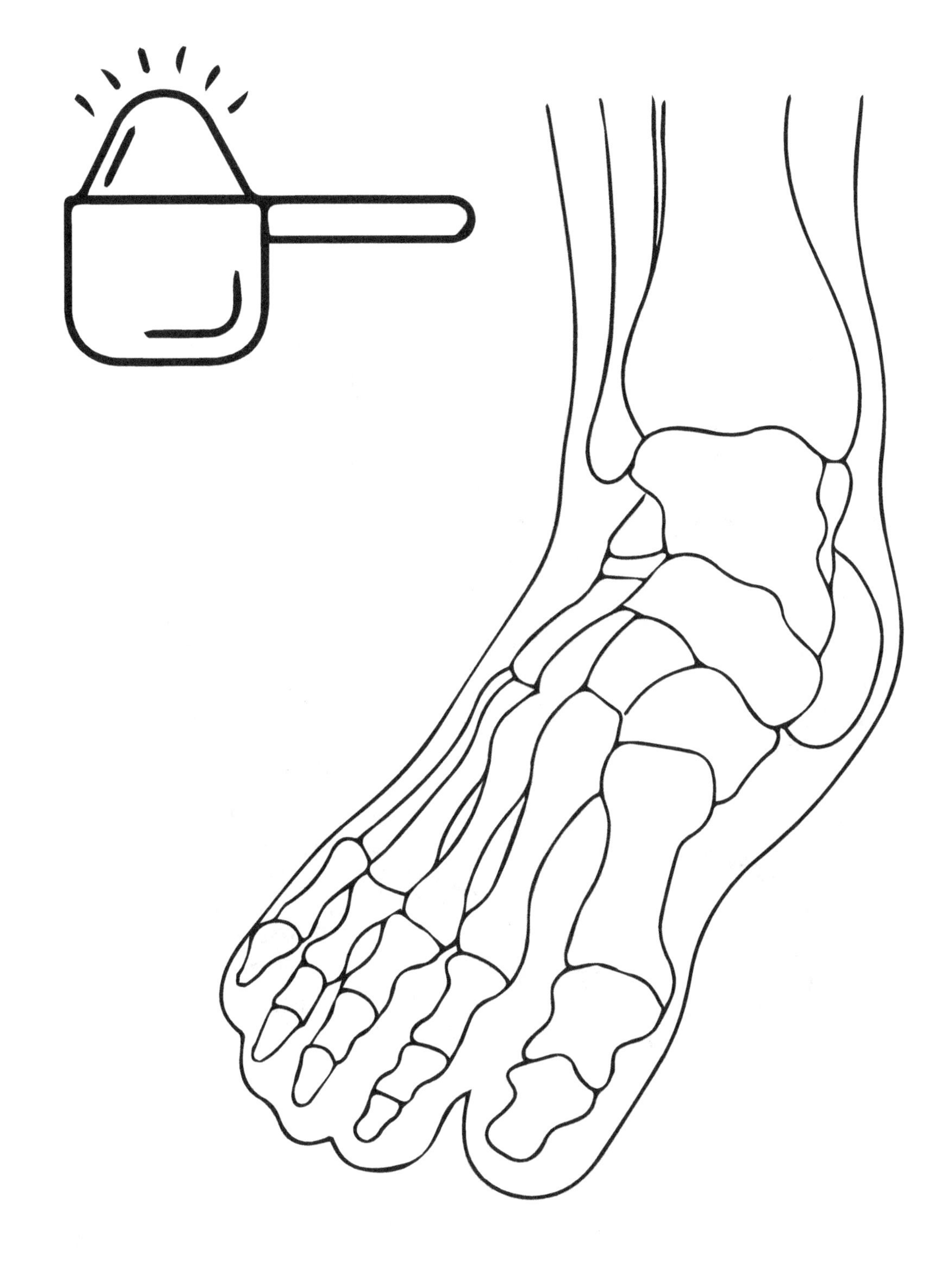

LEGSTRUCTURE

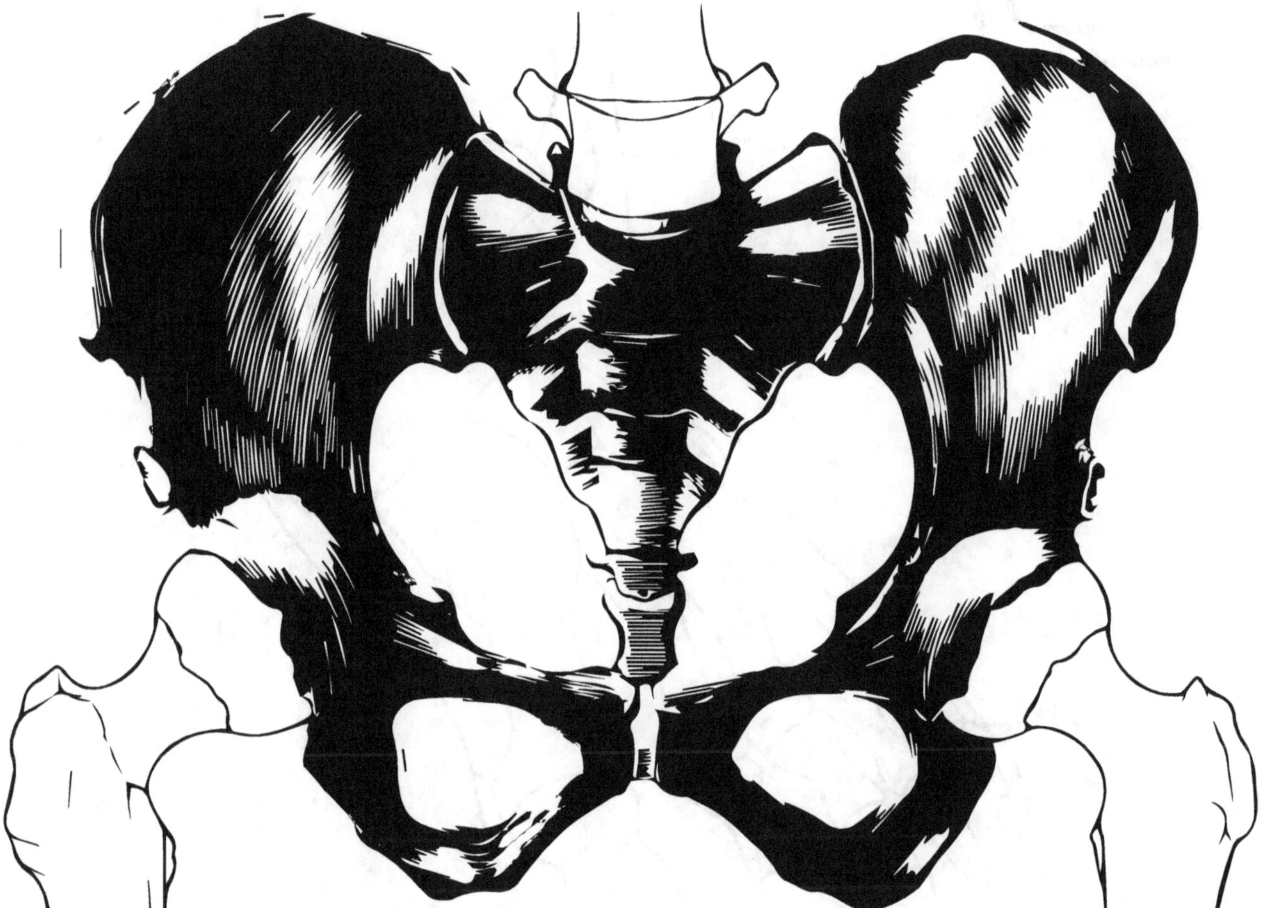

Pelvic bone anatomy

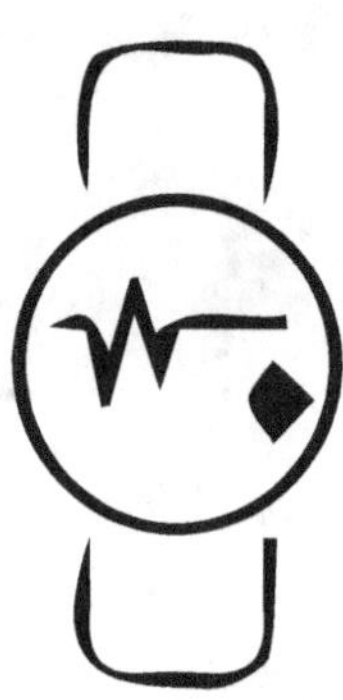